DANCE
AEROBICS

DANCE AEROBICS

BY
MAXINE J. POLLEY

Library of Congress Cataloging in Publication Data

Polley, Maxine.
 Dance Aerobics.

 Includes index.
 1. Aerobic exercises. 2. Dancing. I. Title.
RA781.15.P64   613.7'1   80-23906
ISBN 0-89037-186-5

Anderson World, Inc.
Mountain View, California

Table of Contents

PART ONE: THE FITNESS EXPLOSION 1

        Age Spectrum 4

        Effect on Business 7

        Commercial Sales 9

        Coed Character 11

        The New Concept 12

        Status/Trends 13

        Fat — Who Needs It? 14

        Aerobics 17

        Dance Aerobics 24

PART TWO: CONDUCTING A RECREATIONAL AEROBIC

        DANCE PROGRAM 27

        Behavioral Objectives 32

        Concepts of Recreational Aerobic Dance 32

        Recreational Aerobic Dance Classes 33

        Teaching Suggestions 34

        History of Aerobic Dance 38

        Why Recreational Dance Aerobics Will Live 40

PART THREE:ORIGINAL DANCE AEROBICS ROUTINES 45

        Warm-Up Phase 48

        Stretching 48

        Touch Dancin' 54

        Chocolate Hustle Line Dance 58

        Rockin' Combo 60

        Aerobic Phase 69

        Dance Variety 70

        Navy Special 74

        Aerobic Jog 80

        Aerobic Exercise 82

        Aerobic Flight 88

        Snappy Jazz 94

        Beethovan's Special 99

        Music Box Dancer 107

        Disco Stomp 113

        Cooldown With Nadia 116

        Cooldown With Doctor Z 120

        Summer Cooldown 124

PART FOUR: HELPFUL EXTRAS 130

        Twelve-Week Block Plan 131

        Harvard Step Test 133

        Cardiovascular Efficiency Test 133

        Safety Precautions 136

        Benefits of Total Fitness 140

        1.5 Mile Run Test 145

        Bibliography 147

        About The Author 151

        About The Illustrator 152

Dedication

DANCE AEROBICS
is dedicated to:
my Dad
P.R. McCandless
retired Head of the Science Dept.
Slippery Rock State College
Laboratory School

A man of many accomplishments, is he
Untouched by honors and awards, is he
One of strong convictions and vision
Master of persuasion, encourager of growth
He is a teacher, advisor, and leader.

Acknowledgments

Special thanks:

Kent Austin, an excellent photographer and Christian human being.

Rick Takahashi, a delightful personality and skilled cartoonist.

Rex, Dee, and Dana Polley, my loving, talented, and supportive children.

Introduction

The first section of this book is a bird's-eye view of the fitness explosion—its effects on society, the new concept, and current trends. Cardiovascular fitness is presented via such topics as aerobics, obesity, and physiological changes.

In the next section, the factors involved in planning and carrying out a successful recreational aerobic dance program are outlined and explained.

The inspiration for this handbook came from Ms. Roberta Verley of Northern Michigan University, who was the first to support my earlier efforts. Hopefully, this book will be a major contribution to filling the void in useable aerobic dance materials.

The guiding light for this joyous fitness activity is found in the *Goals for American Recreation.* Since recreation is people-oriented, with a little motivation and experience more leaders will emerge. Aerobic dance has true recreative potential, and can fill increased leisure time with fun, fitness, fellowship and fulfillment. Happy people add to life. They contribute, appreciate and create beauty.

The crux of the book contains fourteen original aerobic dance routines, choreographed specifically for inclusion in the warm-up, aerobic or cooldown phase. As variety is the spice of life, there is something for everyone here—disco, strut, aerobic folk, aerobic exercise, fast locomotor movements, jazz and ballet. A dance potpourri, to be sure.

This book has been written mainly for five groups: 1) junior-senior high school dance and physical education teachers; 2) college recreation, fitness, dance and physical education majors who are preparing to become professional teachers; 3) recreation department leaders and specialists; 4) YMCA/YWCA leaders; 5) commercial sports and health spa instructors.

Record or Cassette ($7.98)
Maxine Polley
Dance Aerobics
P.O. Box 8511
Fort Collins, Colo. 80524
Add 10% for shipping/handling ($1.50 minimum)

Maxine Polley
Metropolitan State College
Denver, Colorado 80204

Part One
The Fitness Explosion

DANCE AEROBICS

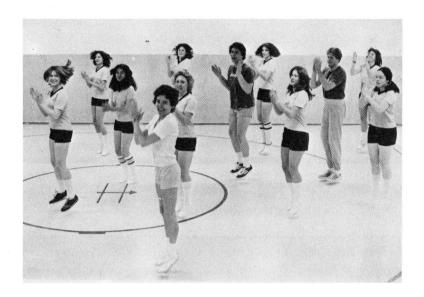

I hear America puffing, the varied exhalations
    I hear.
Those of the joggers, each one risking shinsplints in
    pursuit of transcendental highs.
The iron-pumper grunting as he heaves upon his bench,
    the racquetballer gasping as he strokes.
The health clubber's sigh as he makes ready for the
    Exercycle or slackens his grip upon the Bullworker
    Tensolator.
The delicious panting of the aerobic dancer spinning
    her fantasies to an old show tune.
Puffing with open mouths their strong cardiovascular
    harmonies.

These are the sounds of America shaping up today! The echoing message is that the nation is obsessed with all aspects of fitness, efficiency and youthful vigor.

"There is no question that we are in the midst of a fitness explosion," says George Leonard, author of *The Ultimate Athlete*. "We are discovering that every human being has a God-given right to move efficiently, gracefully and joyfully."

Yes, it has become almost un-American not to exercise. Attribute it to an overdose of "spectatoritis," televised sports

*Source: Matt Clark poem © 1977 by Newsweek. Reprinted by permission. All rights reserved.

or fear of aging and coronary occlusion. Researchers have found that exercise is addictive, and those involved become evangelists who eagerly recruit others.

"We believe that America is going through a physical fitness renaissance that can make a real dent in degenerative diseases, not to mention the quality of life," claims Richard Keelor, director of program development for the President's Council on Physical Fitness and Sports. For the first time in nearly a decade American deaths from cardiovascular disease have fallen below one million. Actuarial standards show that life expectancy has increased two years with men living to 69 and women to 76.7 on the average.

Age Spectrum: No age group is exempt from the great shape-up! In One New York City gym, four hundred children are regularly guided through their gymnastic paces by Susy Prudden, daughter of the pioneer exercise authority Bonnie Prudden. "A child actually develops fifty percent of its physical potential by the age of three," explains the teacher. Not only in New York, but also in Southern California and Colorado the "kiddie fit" movement is widespread.

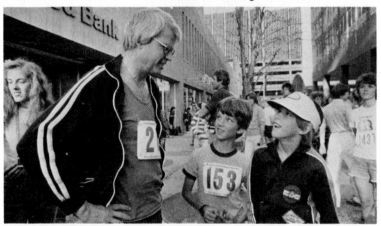

Kids competing in age-group running is relatively new. *Runner's World* Magazine counts at least 20,000 children in the Road Runners Club of America's Age-Group Championships. The best of the boys have run a sub-five minute mile at age eleven, under 4:20 by age fifteen. The top girls have gone below five minutes at thirteen, under 4:50 by fifteen. "Olympic times are coming down so fast," says chairman Barry Geisler, "that if you want to become a world-class runner, there is no question that you're going to have to run age-group."

Competing among themselves, the "Skip-Its" from Douglass Elementary School in Boulder, Colorado, have achieved national rope-skipping honors. As Mr. Rich Cendali proclaims, "There is no better way to relate to kids than through kids themselves." Besides performing for schools, service organizations, state and national Health, Physical Education, Recreation and Dance conventions, they have skipped for N.B.C. Newsreel, performed on the steps of the Capital in Washington, D.C. and on international television in "Teachers Around the World," produced by Fuji Telecasting Com-

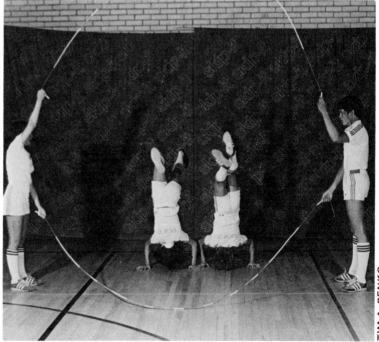

pany, Tokyo, Japan. The "Skip-Its" are listed in the *Guinness Book of World Records* for jumping a 100-foot jump-rope with fifty-one children, completing six jumps.

Last year, JOPER cited a pilot program called the Health Hustle, initiated at the same time every day in eighty elementary schools in Scarborough, Ontario. For twelve minutes, while music came over the PA system, the students, the principal, teachers, secretaries and the janitor exercised to disco rhythms. Improved discipline, schoolwork, attentiveness, plus an overall "great feeling" resulted. The Health

Hustle concept is spreading rapidly.

At the other end of the spectrum, many senior citizens in nursing homes now exercise while sitting or standing, to the catchy beat of disco music. Not exempt from jogging, seniors lope along amidst the runners. They don't want anyone feeding them with a spoon or carrying them to the bathroom. They know the only way to keep mobility is by maintaining strength and endurance.

Joggers of all ages in motion, that's the most visible sign of the fitness boom. The indoor track at Boston's main Y.M.C.A. has grown so crowded you have to run in step, or you'll get killed. "They take over the streets on weekends, sometimes one hundred strong, five and six abreast and refuse to get out of traffic lanes," complains the city manager of Los Altos Hills, California.

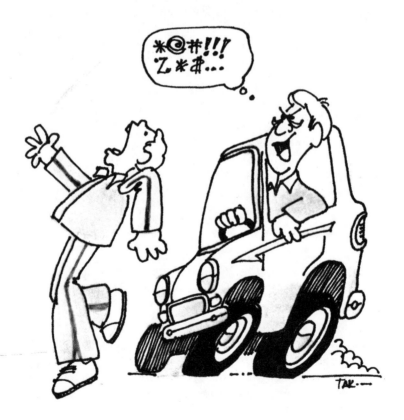

The ranks of the joggers, which includes an army of runners, have been swelled by the nation's fifty million tennis freaks. These racquet buffs have belatedly discovered that they must "get in shape to play, rather than play to get in shape." However, the very popular newcomer called racquetball boasts a growing 10.6 million adherents according to the A.C. Neilson Survey covering 1976 to 1979. Experts say the rationale for its immediate success is that you can learn enough racquetball fundamentals to start enjoying yourself within five minutes.

Effect on Business: The benefits of exercise are being recognized by private industry, which loses an estimated fifty-four million dolars to common backaches in lost output each year. "The typical job in the modern office or auto-

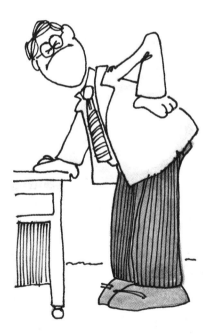

mated factory requires less physical exertion than a hot shower," states Richard Keelor of the Presidents Council on Physical Fitness and Sports.

Some one hundred fifty companies, members of the American Association of Fitness Directors in Business and Industry (AAFDBI) have active programs. About fifty more are organizing them. These programs vary across the country. At Pepsico and Wausau Insurance, some one thousand employees are involved. Prudential provides several different programs—some open to executives only, others for all employees. Kimberly-Clark requires extensive testing before and after activity. The Johnson & Johnson effort is part of a larger comprehensive health promotion program called "Live for Life," including three thousand five hundred employees. Flex time, cost-effective models, mandatory stress tests, compliance, closet exercisers, and PEP have become common terms. Unlike scientists, business people don't wait until all the evidence is in, to make a decision.

Key executives boost productivity by participating in fitness programs. Today's junior executive is encouraged to set off for work an hour or so early, toting a squash racket, or to skip the two-martini lunch for some laps across the Y.M.C.A. pool. In fact, Hospital Corporation of America pays employees sixty-four cents a swimming mile beyond required minimums. The executive's secretary is probably enrolled in some form of slimnastics. Chances are that his wife is into the newest wrinkle, aerobic dance—rhythmic, dance-inspired movements done to music.

Profit entrepreneurs who monitor the nation's leisure-time pulse seem convinced that the fitness urge is embedding itself in the American psyche as indelibly as it did in ancient Greece. "Fitness is being encouraged by the fear of social isolation, if one is not involved in physical activity," observes psychologist and author Dr. Richard Suinn, Colorado State University.

One of the most elaborate of the physical fitness programs now under way in some three thousand corporations is that run by Chase Manhattan Bank in New York City. The bank operates a cardiovascular fitness laboratory for four hundred of its executives, who get lectures on heart disease along with exercise. In time, their amount of body fat and oxygen consumption drops. Rockwell International has extensive recreation centers at some facilities. The oldest, at El Segunda, California, has sixteen acres with a gym, rifle range, six tennis courts and two lighted softball diamonds. "Losing weight is secondary to fitness," says manager Ken White. Some sixty-year-olds who exercise have proven to be in better shape than some in their mid-twenties who don't.

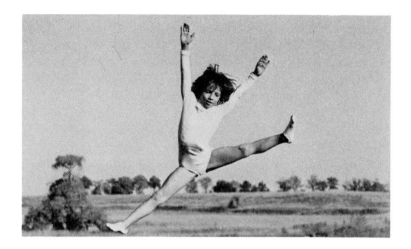

Forney Engineering Company, near Dallas, is typical of smaller firms that have no fancy facilities but do support active health programs. The firm, which laid out a one-mile walking route and built a quarter-mile dirt track, will spend ten thousand dollars on their program this year.

Those large companies lacking exercise facilities in their headquarters are turning to outside specialists. Fitness Systems, Inc., in Los Angeles, provides exercise programs to businesses. After six months in this program, executives have usually improved by thirty percent in cardiovascular conditions. Most lose three and one-half pounds of pure fat. Also gone are the old topics of cars and women in some male conversations, being supplanted by physical fitness topics such as 'the best shoes or running times.'

Commercial Sales: Catering to fitness has become a booming business. The National Sporting Goods Association reports annual sales of well over sixteen billion dollars. The marriage of fashion and fitness is hardly new. Sales of tennis togs alone have passed three hundred million a year. A tennis outfit is almost like a face lift, making a woman look younger whether she actually plays or not! The high-fashion jogger dons a fleece-knit or velour track suit with rugbyesque stripes before making his rounds. Five years ago, running shoes were made exclusively for men. Now, with some one hundred models for women, manufacturers are trying to keep pace with the astronomical demands.

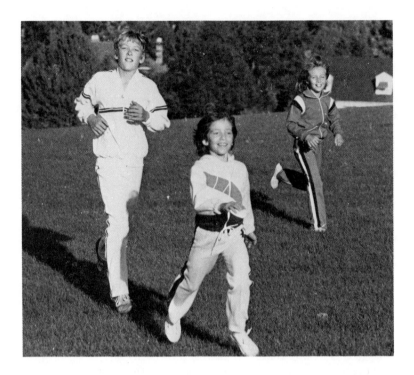

All this massive expenditure of energy is fueling a two bil-lion-dollar-a-year supply industry. Americans now shell out more than sixty-five million dollars annually for home-condi-tioning equipment. Beyond this, Nautilus exercise equip-ment, originally developed for the medical and athletic com-munity, has been sold to more than four hundred condition-ing centers within six years. Ed Farnham, the general mana-ger, reports, "Orders are in a state of geometric progression, I see no letup." Enrollment in health spas is up twenty-five percent from last year, while sales of health foods have reached well beyond the organic cult. Stow-Mills, the largest health-food distributor in New England, says that it is selling no less than twelve tons of granola each month. Even the humble sport of rope-jumping is on the upswing. Bobby Hinds re-ports some seventy thousand orders a month for his nylon-and-plastic Lifeline jump-ropes.

"You would have to run four eight-minute miles to get the benefit of ten minutes of consistent rope-jumping," contends Hinds.

Every national craze requires its how-to manuals, thus the publishing industry is working overtime. There are no fewer than one thousand and eight hundred books on fitness

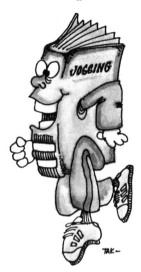

and health currently in print. If the movement has a Bible, it is Dallas physician Kenneth Cooper's 1968 book, *Aerobics.* His first three books on aerobics have sold six million copies. Many bookstores report that James Fixx's second book is selling nearly as fast as his first one.

Runner's World Magazine has become one of the success stories of publishing. Considered the monthly Bible of runners in the United States, the magazine founded on a shoestring sixteen years ago has seen circulation zoom from 35,200 in 1975 to over 400,000 in 1980. Publisher Bob Anderson and his wife, Rita, are now the owners of a growing empire of separate companies specializing in running books, magazines, films, library services and a mail-order house for runners and other athletes.

Coed Character: Perhaps the most salient aspect of shaping up is its new coed character. Women first began invading the tennis courts in droves after Billie Jean King demolished Bobby Riggs on television in 1973. Since then, the feminization of fitness has taken a pervasive hold. The sexual integration of the fitness scene is gradually transforming the solitary agony of keeping fit into a social activity. Commercial sports preserves have replaced the singles bar as the most popular "meet-market." To go out on jogging dates is becoming increasingly popular. It's a very normal thing, since running is an easy way to get to know someone.

New Concept: According to the Y's national director of Health and Physical Education, Lloyd Arnold, fitness used to mean flexibility, endurance, strength and power. Now the crux is endurance or cardiovascular efficiency. Super-strong is not synonymous with healthy. The thread running through the aerobics concept is to gain a training effect via rhythmic exercise done for twenty to thirty minutes, while staying within the target zone. Dr. Ken Cooper, the aerobics pioneer, has scientifically quantified exercise by means of a pharmacopoeia. Says Dr. Cooper, "Those who are serious about exercise usually end up running."

On the other side of the hill, former Olympian Dick Taylor of Devil's Thumb Ranch cries, "Forget great goals! Suppose you say, well, if I do another quarter of a mile each week or I'm going to run a mile in 6:18 or something, so what? Unburdened by great goals, women basically want self-acceptance." Taylor carries the torch high for rhythm running—for the fun of it! By using a gentle run, then going back to a race-walk, then long "Farmer Brown" strides, he prevents beginners from experiencing negative aspects such as pain. He says his motivation is simply that it feels nice to move through the woods. "It's very satisfying, it's very gracefully sensual; it's just pleasurable." Having gotten people to run at his ranch, Taylor says he has another problem. People run too much, thinking that they have to run every day like brushing their teeth. What could be more grim than brushing your teeth? Most people have this compulsion about habits that are supposed to be good for you. Three times a week is fine, he says.

Rewards of running are ageless. Of a divided circle representing the human being, half represents strength, the other half frailty—uncertainty, says Taylor. In other words, what's in front of you, the part of yourself that you don't know, is the mystery. Frailty becomes a fascination that ultimately pulls the runner along. In a protected sort of way, the individual drifts back and forth.

Having run in three road races, Taylor expressed a feeling of exhilaration running among two thousand runners. The rationale he cited was "the genuine elemental sharing of a total human situation. What draws these masses of people together is not how healthy they are, but how human they are—that is, mortal. That's what they share."

STATUS AND TRENDS

The Harris Perrier Survey of Fitness in America (done for the French mineral water firm that co-sponsors the New York marathon and other races) is based on personal interviews with one thousand five hundred ten people and a telephone sample of one hundred eighty runners. Findings show that forty-one percent of Americans do not exercise, forty-four percent are somewhat active, and only fifteen percent are seriously involved in regular exercise. This latter group of fitness freaks tends to favor calisthenics, running and basketball, while those who are less committed to physical exertion favor bowling, walking and swimming. On the basis of the poll, Harris sees a bright future for calisthenics, softball and basketball. There will be a slow rise or a decline for tennis, bowling, bicycling, hiking and swimming. Other findings include:

1. Americans who exercise more or less regularly smoke as much as those who do not.

2. In the past two years more women than men have taken up some form of exercise for the first time.

3. Some eighty-two percent of parents want their daughters to take up sports and exercise, almost as many as those who favor physical activity for their sons (eighty-nine percent).

4. The family is "one of the most important but overlooked influences" on physical fitness; children tend to take up sports if their parents do.

5. For boys as well as girls, football is one of the top two physical activities that parents oppose for their children. Wrestling is most opposed for girls, boxing for the boys.

6. Some twenty-eight percent of highly active Americans say that exercise has improved their sex life, "a claim," admits Harris, "we could not check out in this study."

Source: ©1978 by Newsgroup Publications, Inc. Reprinted by permission of *New York Magazine.*

Harris presents a mixed future for physical fitness. Enthusiasm for exercise is on the rise, but a grumbling resistance to the trend is also digging in. John Van Doorn calls it the intimidation by a new class, the "physical elite." Standard forms of elitism were breeding, money, intellect or attachment to swift-moving fads in politics and fashion. This new elite class exercises, which is guilt-inducing to the rest of us. The idea of a super-race is intimidating. Today's bizarre behavior by a small band of runners may be tomorrow's norm for millions.

FAT-WHO NEEDS IT?

America's weight woes grow. More than half the population is overweight (ten percent over the desired weight),

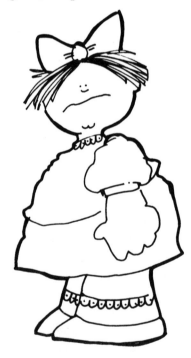

according to Metropolitan Life Insurance Company figures. The struggle against flab is not only uphill but getting steeper all the time.

The best way to tell if you are overweight is by measuring

your percent of body fat via skinfold thickness using a caliper. This is standard procedure in adult fitness programs. Acceptable levels as suggested by Dr. Kenneth Cooper are: for men, less than nineteen percent, for women, less than twenty-two percent. Athletes should be under fifteen percent.

Studies have shown that youngsters who are fat as children tend to be fat as adults. Obese children need exercise even more than other youngsters. Early onset of obesity results in a marked increase in the total number of fat cells. Instead of the usual adult number, twenty-five to thirty billion fat cells, the total may reach one hundred billion. If physical activity is increased in early life, however, the final number of fat cells will be less or undetectable.

Adult onset obesity is the most common form. It is characterized by an increase in size, rather than number of existing fat cells. Weight is gained because the caloric intake of the food exceeds that used in daily activity. To lose weight, reverse the process—take in fewer calories, or burn more.

By using a standard calorie chart, estimate your daily food intake. If you are a normally active person, the basic number of calories it takes to maintain your present weight can be determined by multiplying your weight in pounds times fifteen; sedentary people use twelve, pregnant or lactating mothers should, advises Dr. Cooper, multiply by eighteen. If your caloric intake is much more than this total figure, you will gain weight. If much below, you will start losing weight.

How much can you safely lose and how fast? An example of an unhealthy effort at becoming healthy is to go from appalling overeating to compulsive smoking to a saccharin-kick diet to a two-week fast on liquid protein. According to the Food and Drug Administration, you could be technically dead. But like those characters in Faulkner, you will endure. Dr. Kenneth Cooper recommends losing two pounds per week, as a safe realistic approach. This means one thou-sand calories a day, since one pound represents three thousand five hundred calories. When weight is lost slowly, the body has time to adapt to the new eating pattern.

If a person fasts (goes without food for days), however,

lean body mass or muscle is also lost. Sometimes as much as one-half to two-thirds of the weight lost is not fat but lean body mass. Appetite suppressants, especially amphetamines, should not be used because of their temporary effect and potential danger. Follow your doctor's guidelines. He will probably put you on a one-a-day multiple vitamin and mineral supplement when consuming fewer than one thousand calories per day. Remember to stay away from food fads and problem foods such as refined sugars, coffee (not more than two or three cups a day), tea, colas and alcohol. Yes, as the old adage goes: Everything I like is either illegal, immoral or fattening.

Meg Greenfield claims that the two most fattening things she knows are remorse and self-pity—each of them good for at least another thousand calorie shot. The happy fat person is a myth. Fat is misery. Obese workers (twenty percent over the desired weight) are losing out on pay raises, promotions, and jobs. A California survey of one thousand patients showed that more than fourteen percent could not get a job due to their weight. The problem is worsening as more and more Americans add too many pounds. Seen as second-class citizens job-wise, they are discriminated against. Some tortoise-shaped individuals tell of losing social status and self-esteem, of being denied a promotion or being fired, simply because they are overweight. The consensus is that the boss wants good-looking women around the office.

As for research, nearly a decade ago R.D. Myers established a correspondence between the amount of sodium, calcium, magnesium and potassium to body temperature and feeding. It was discovered that if the level of calcium in the brain increases and the level of sodium remains the same, there is a drop in body temperature and an increase in eating. This ratio is thought to comprise an organism's weight "set-point." It acts as a thermostat, being set just before or after birth. The set-point determines what the optimum amount of food for a particular organism should be by specifying the "operating temperature." Overeating for you may be just right for someone else. Everyone has a specific pre-set weight balance which must be maintained. Fad diets don't change one's set-point. Regulating your energy balance is needed, not starving yourself. Weight change must be done by altering the set-point and allowing your body to adjust to the new level.

The food ratio recommended by the American Heart Association is fourteen percent protein, thirty-five percent fat, and fifty-one percent carbohydrates. In general, cut down on the amount, not the type of food eaten. Dr. Michael Lakat states that each person's set-point is pre-determined and specific to that person, just like intelligence or hair color. Food intake is subsequently dependent upon it. Weight thus determines eating, eating does not determine weight.

AEROBICS

Some thirty million Americans are running religiously, to save their lives—in essence, the quality of life itself. Yes, through technology, years have been added to life, but has life been added to years? Why should life seem over when housewives get their kids into school? Should men lose their independence to machines and paperwork, becoming mere robots? Need senior citizens be spoon fed and carried from one place to another? For them, strength and mobility mean independence.

Americans are waking up! We are beginning to assert our God-given right to be totally fit. We want and shall have cardiovascular efficiency (heart and lungs) and youthful vigor. See the aerobic "glow" that comes after exercise—that time when the circulation is humming and you feel so awake and alive! Total fitness means that all three entities, the mind, body and spirit, are in top shape. Yes, the holistic concept of health has been revived.

The focus is now on preventive medicine. Responsibility for health or total fitness has been placed back on the individual's shoulders where it belongs. For too long we have been completely dependent upon the medical profession. As Dr. Kenneth Cooper, the aerobics pioneer says, "Ours is a medical system which meets the patient when he is already diseased...and when no matter how sophisticated the treatment, very little can be done to relieve his disability or extend his life."

Dr. Kenneth Cooper promoted the right idea at the right time—right for a sedentary society whose number one killer is heart disease. A former Air Force physician, Dr. Cooper appropriated the term "aerobics" to describe his exercise program to strengthen the heart, lungs and blood vessels. Since his first book, *Aerobics* (1968) was published, he has ridden the crest of the physical fitness revolution. In the ensuing nine years he wrote *The New Aerobics*, and with his wife Mildred's input, co-authored *Aerobics for Women*. Together these three volumes have sold six million copies.

"Physical fitness is more than letting your fingers walk through the yellow pages," says Erma Bombeck. "True physical fitness is a function of endurance—how long one can continue exercising before becoming exhausted," cites Dr. Cooper. Since endurance is a function of how well one utilizes oxygen, he evaluates exercise by its effect on the cardiovascular system. Dr. Cooper catalogued popular forms of exercise into measurable amounts. Through his aerobic point system, exercise is continuously quantified. As readers of Cooper's books know, a female of any age can accumulate her necessary minimal twenty-four points a week (thirty for males) by running, walking, swimming, cycling or by doing other aerobic exercise four or five times a week. For example, cycling two miles in six minutes is worth three points. Running a seven-minute mile is worth five points. Run that five times a week and your heart and lungs should stay in good condition. It is desirable to earn more points, of course. Points are based on intensity and duration of exercise. Cooper rates cross-country skiing and swimming ahead of running as the best cardiovascular activities. These also have the least risk of muscular and skeletal injury. He puts bicycling and walking in fourth and fifth places. If the exercise is vigorous enough to produce a sustained heart rate of one hundred fifty beats per minute or more, positive conditioning effects begin after five minutes.

In contrast, isometric activities are not aerobic. Such exertions as weight-lifting and push-ups strengthen the muscles, causing them to constrict, thus narrowing the blood vessels and reducing blood circulation. For those with a tendency toward high blood pressure, isometrics can be hazardous.

Aerobic activities tax the heart and lungs sufficiently when they are done vigorously for twenty minutes, staying within the individual's target zone. "If you want to maintain your present physical fitness level, exercise twice a week. To improve, do aerobic exercise three times a week, on alternate days. To change body composition or lose weight around the middle, exercise four times a week," explains Dr. Max Morton, CSU's director of Adult Fitness and Cardiac Rehabilitation. "Caution and common sense must prevail when beginning any conditioning program," states Sports Medicine physician Dr. John Harvey of Fort Collins.

What is the talked-about twelve-minute test? These are Cooper's field tests involving walking and running on a level surface, or just walking, swimming, or cycling. You cover the greatest distance that you can in twelve minutes. Dr. Cooper WARNS us—"be in condition prior to taking any test." Warm-up before and cool-down properly afterwards. According to your age and test score, you will be categorized into one of the five classes ranging from very poor to excellent. Tested then, will be your VO2 max without treadmills or expired gas collectors.

For grading purposes in high school or college, twelve-minute test scores, total miles run, the mile and one-half classifications, etc., are helpful. Some charts can be used for a pre-and post-test to show improvement in total fitness. Yes, Dr. Ken Cooper has taken the guesswork out of exercise. Educators should be quick to employ his scientific data.

Mrs. Kenneth Cooper, in *Aerobics* for Women, tells women: "You can't store up physical fitness; there simply isn't a layaway plan. Exercise is something you have to make up your mind to do daily or every other day. Stop-and-start conditioning has no value whatever, in building up your aerobic capacity (the best index of overall physical fitness). In fact, it can be harmful. Turning a light switch on and off does more to deplete the bulb's lasting power than letting it burn; on-again, off-again exercise is also an unsatisfactory way to prolong endurance."

Bodies at rest tend to remain at rest, states the law of inertia. Per-Orlof Astrand, the noted Swedish physiologist, feels it is much more dangerous to be inactive than active. Americans who don't exercise are probably in worse shape than ever, according to Dr. Warren Guild, former president of the American College of Sports Medicine. Middle age begins when people have been out of college or the armed forces for three years. It used to begin when you were forty. Maturational kinesiologists agree that physical fitness postpones degradation or the onset of aging. This is the major reason why kinesiologists claim that participation in aerobic activities must be started at an early age, and maintained. Physical fitness efforts pay off handsomely. At the first National Conference on Physical Fitness and Sports, the recent drop in the nation's mortality rate and increases in life expectancy were credited to improved exercise habits. The nation has seen a one percent per year drop in the incidence of fatal heart disease.

Not only through research, but also by example, Dr. Cooper provides leadership. Tennis and swimming are his most frequent forms of aerobic exercise. Regardless of what country Dr. Ken Cooper is in, he runs three miles daily. Once a pudgy, two hundred pound medical student, he admits he doesn't like running three miles every day, but if he stops he deteriorates. "The only excuses for not exercising regularly are sickness, immunization, all-out fatigue, extremes of temperature or weather and blessed events," Mrs. Cooper proclaims.

Jogging along with aerobic dance is beneficial. Both are addicting. Jackie Sorensen reports that ninety percent or more of the women who take aerobic dancing classes sign up for another session. Many joggers build from fifteen to fifty miles of running a week. A few progress on toward the one-hundred-mile a week mark. Dr. Thomas Bassler of the Centinela Valley Community Hospital in California and president of the American Medical Joggers Association (a one-thousand-member group of running M.D.s), has run in sixty-six marathons and done three thousand autopsies. Bassler believes that anyone who has ever reached the level of physical training that will enable him to finish a marathon is permanently immune to heart attack. Dr. Cooper's Annual Tyler Cup Invitational draws some one hundred sixty top corporation executives from about sixteen different states to compete in eight two-mile heats. This competition is held on Dr. Cooper's eleven acre garden paradise estate in north Dallas. When Dr. Cooper says that his aerobics is "an idea that could reshape the lives of millions," you begin to believe him.

Dr. Meyer Friedman cites Type-A behavior pattern as the prime factor in heart disease found in young adults. This pattern is displayed by individuals showing consistent aggressiveness, impatience, excessive competitive drive and a sense of time urgency. They also frequently exhibit a free-floating form of hostility. The Type-A person at first rises to any challenge. He tries hard to control a highly stressful situation, but when his best efforts fail, he feels helpless and his attempts to master it suffer more than Type-B individuals. Life's tragedies are particularly dangerous for the Type-A person. Stress increases the production of blood cholesterol, plus adrenalin and noradrenalin which results in high blood pressure. (Above one hundred forty over ninety is considered high, with hypertension defined as above one hundred sixty over ninety-five).

The American lifestyle fosters high blood pressure (the major cause of strokes) in one out of every three Americans. Stress keeps the body in a state of tension, rather than allowing it to relax properly. However, exercise holds the adrenal hormones in balance, relaxation is forthcoming, the mind and body become satisfied. Aerobic exercise acts as an antidepressant. Psychic benefits have inspired a San Diego psychiatrist to put together a program which he calls "running therapy." After personally discovering its purgative powers a few years ago, Dr. Thaddeus Kostrubala decided to begin running with patients who were not progressing. His initial group included a heroin addict, a paranoid, a mental depressive and a potential suicide. By setting a pace that encouraged each patient to talk comfortably, major positive personality changes did, in fact, occur.

Joggers claim to have been cured of every ill from insomnia to impotence. Those possessing the stamina for close to an hour of steady running, report an altered state of consciousness, a sudden rush of perceptive powers coupled with an almost Zen-like peace. Some call it a hormonal high—their confessional, wailing wall, or psychiatric couch. Runners claim the feeling that nobody can touch you and you're the greatest—a positive self-concept, so important in a healthy personality. This beautiful sensation of movement usually takes over after a runner has built up enough endurance so that he can run effortlessly for an hour. Dr. William Glasser, psychiatrist and author, describes this feeling of euphoria as PA or positive addiction, best achieved through running.

A 1976 report from the Mayo Clinic stated that, of heart patients actively involved in an exercise program, "all (the test subjects) had....an increase in self-esteem and a more positive attitude toward their work and their disability." A study at Purdue University showed that those who progressed from a "least-fit" level achieved increased emotional stability, imagination, self-assurance, besides self-sufficiency.

According to the American Heart Association, forty percent of fatal heart attacks come without warning. A study presented to the American Heart Association by Dr. Ralph Paffenbarger of the University of California at Berkeley shows that strenuous exercise can prevent heart attacks. He studied seventeen thousand male alumni of Harvard, age thirty-five to seventy-four, for a decade. His conclusion: The protective effect of being active seemed to hold, regardless of whether the men had other serious risk factors such as cigarette smoking, high blood pressure, parental heart attacks or lack of athletic experience.

Cardiologists agree that the more physically fit individual has a better chance of surviving a heart attack and recovery is quicker. Dr. Terrence Kavanaugh, medical director of the Toronto Cardiac Rehabilitation Center, reports a 1.4 percent-per-annum mortality rate from 1967-1976 for cardiacs who exercised, compared to six to twelve percent for non-exercisers. This data resulted from seven hundred eighty patients, probably the largest exercise coronary rehabilitation group in the world.

Of the three thousand plus people who turned out to run a marathon in Honolulu, Hawaii last year, more than one hundred runners had previously suffered heart attacks or had prior coronary problems.

Lenore R. Zohman, M.D., one of the most famous exercise cardiologists in the world, has successfully used aerobic dance in cardiac rehabilitation. A widely traveled lecturer and frequent television guest, Dr. Zohman obtained her M.D. degree at Downstate Medical Center in her native New York City and then spent ten years in advanced cardiology training. In 1962 she developed, and continues to direct, the Cardiopulmonary Rehabilitation Program at Montefiore Hospital and Medical Center in New York City, the major teaching hospital of the Albert Einstein College of Medicine.

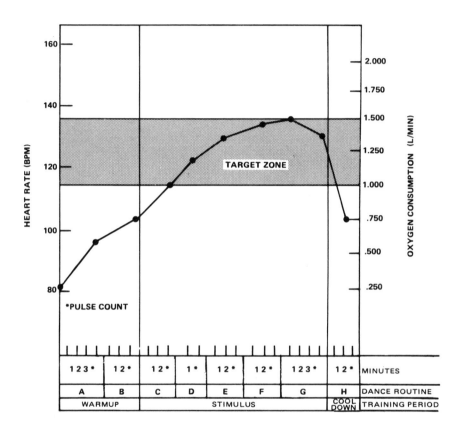

According to Zohman and Kattus, "fitness dancing puts the joints of the body through their range of motion; exercises muscles of the extremities, trunk and neck; and provides a type of interval training for the cardiovascular system. As shown, the warm-up consists of easier routines, a stimulus period of the more demanding ones, and a cool-down later. Nobody drops out—even cardiac patients, since the stimulus period particularly, can be scaled down to low or moderate intensity and need not be taken in high gear.* The energy cost of low-level dancing is metabolically similar to that of walking, medium intensity to that of playing tennis, and high intensity to that of playing hockey. Fitness dancing will produce a training effect since heart rates reach the target zone, as shown."

DANCE AEROBICS

There is still one question unanswered scientifically. Does running add years to your life? According to today's actuarial standards, if you exercise regularly, you'll gain four years.

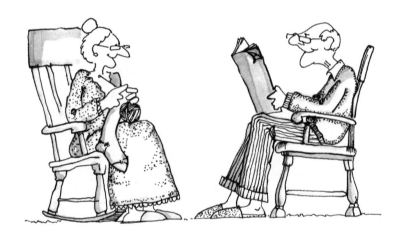

*Low-level dancing cost 3.96 Cal/min for the women and 4.17 Cal/min for the men. Medium-level came out to 6.28 for the women and 6.86 for the men, and high required 7.75 for women and 9.48 for men (Data for Aerobic Dancing specifically).

Scientific data resulting from ongoing studies at Cooper's Aerobic Center, involving longevity, and jogging will be available sometime in the 1980s. However, a woman jogger makes a point: "I don't care how long I live, just so I LIVE!"

In Dr. Cooper's most recent book, *The Aerobics Way,* he muses over the past decade with satisfaction. Life spans have increased. The national death rate from heart disease has dropped almost fourteen percent. He is optimistic about America's future. Winston Churchill said it best: "The farther backward you can look, the farther forward you are likely to see."

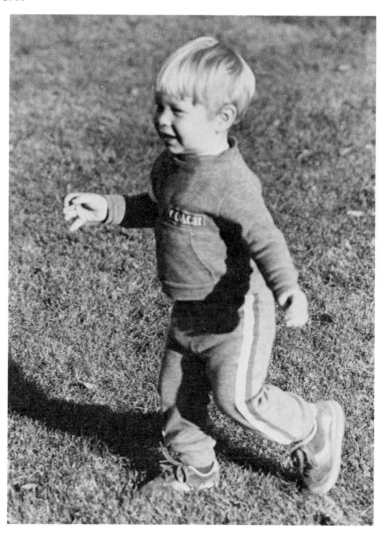

Part Two
Conducting a Recreational Dance Aerobics Group Program

If a man does not know to what port he is sailing, no wind is favorable.

—Socrates

The greatest personal defeat of man is the difference between what he is capable of becoming and what, in fact, he became.

—Ashley Montagu

To use leisure intelligently and profitably is the final test of civilization.

—Jay B. Nash

You ought not to attempt to cure the eyes without the head, or the head without the body...the body without the soul...for the part can never be well unless the whole is well.

—Plato, 399 B.C.

The dance aerobics program is recreational. It should be conducted and accepted in the light of the following Goals for American Recreation.

1. **Personal Fulfillment.** Recreation means more than mere play. Participation and achievement in challenging recreational activities will help to narrow the gap between the individual's potentialities and his or her accomplishments. Early success experiences without stressful competition, in an uplifting social atmosphere, will enhance the individual's self-concept and he or she will feel good about themselves and others.

2. **Democratic Human Relations.** The dignity and worth of each individual should be enhanced through vocational and avocational activities. By cooperating for the common good, obeying the law, showing behavior based on high ethical standards and genuine concern for the welfare of others, democracy will live.

3. **Leisure Skills and Interests.** "Leisure, a by-product of man's conquest of nature, is a gift of man's creative genius," states Dr. Max Shirley, chairman of recreation, University of Northern Colorado. "Life has become easier, yielding more of both true and forced leisure time, but the boredom of automated existence and the frustration of job displacement is apparent. Good use of leisure time became an established Principle of Education in 1918. No longer a work society, sociologists say that the true meaning of life can be found in the people's leisure." Accordingly, during free or unobligated time, individuals will repeat what they enjoy, according to the "pleasure principle." To experience that joy, some degree of skill is essential. An effective leader will not only teach skills but will reinforce the individual's choice of leisure activities, being especially supportive of lifetime sports and hobbies. Leisure activities must make up for jobs that are too small for our spirit.

4. **Health and Fitness.** Our nation is just as strong as its people. Regrettably, the "don't walk" light on busy street corners has become a sign of our times. Activity is no longer required for basic survival. However, nature tends to eliminate those who have relinquished their functional usefulness. Unfortunately, nature does not appear to favor mind over matter.

Technology has provided "things" but only temporary happiness. "Things" produced by mere robots are inadequate substitutes for health and fitness.

Presently, our sedentary nation as a whole is experiencing a growth of "collective awareness." A strong motivating force from within is hungry for health and happiness. Having lost faith in much of society—government, business, marriage, the church and so on—people are turning to themselves, putting what faith they can muster into their own body temples, says James Fixx. With more leisure time on their hands, some are listening to or testing the testimonials of athletes.

As the need for aerobic activities increases, effective recreational leaders can cheerfully provide attractive vehicles for significant human health and fitness endeavors.

5. **Creative Expression and Aesthetic Appreciation.** Beauty is its own excuse for being. All agree there is much beauty in movement and expression, with the ultimate in human expression being creativity. In essence, creativity represents the very core of human uniqueness. It parallels hope, and will sustain life when all else fails. Thus, personal expression, creative experience and aesthetic appreciation give depth and richness to life.

6. **Environment for Living in a Leisure Society.** The environment will be enriched in direct proportion to the health and fitness of its people. Those who would conserve the deep-seated human values of recreation must conserve also the phenomena of nature. Controlling the character of the environment means more than setting aside land for the full enjoyment and development of a people's leisure. The finer cultural proclivities of a civilized people require an artistic environment suitable to the performing arts. The quality of life in America is on a steady rise toward higher goals, which in a leisure society is reflected in the recreation of the people.

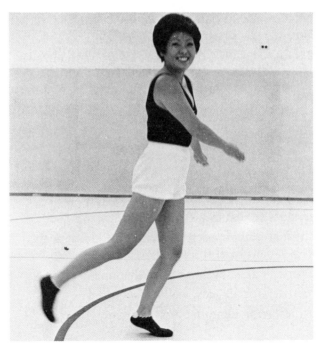

BEHAVIORAL OBJECTIVES
FOR RECREATIONAL DANCE AEROBICS

Upon completion of this dance aerobics program students should be able to:

1. Show a joyful appreciation for the dance aerobics activity.

2. Know that he or she has become more physically fit; some may even lose weight.

3. Be knowledgeable concerning basic fitness information.

4. Execute fifteen routines on the secondary level while following the instructor's lead.

5. Create and demonstrate a short dance aerobics routine if desired.

Concept of Recreational Dance Aerobics

Recreational dance aerobics consists of several series of specially choreographed routines which combine jogging with rhythmic dance movements to music.

The chief objectives are *fun, fitness, fellowship* and *fulfillment.* With a few modifications, individuals from six to sixty can enjoy this innovative recreational activity. Immediate success, excellent leadership, and the constant challenge of new routines to catchy rhythms keeps the activity ever exciting and satisfying.

Recreational dance aerobics is a complete physical fitness program in itself. As has been said about fitness, it is like a viable banking system; you put in deposits of unrestrained body movements and dancing, and withdraw such dividends as muscle tone, balance and coordination, plus greater cardiovascular (heart and lung) efficiency.

Dance aerobics is an extremely attractive alternative to many other training practices. Advantages include:

- a group activity; the social dimension
- individual fitness levels; a walk, jog or run pace
- individual preference; elevation of kicks, leaps, hops as well as height of arm movements
- the focus; participation rather than memorization
- an activity for all ages, walking required
- routines, choreographed for everyone

- great variety of steps, great variety of routines
- an escape from boredom; mental and physical challenge
- has the potential for developing grace, poise, and rhythm
- an all-weather activity, indoors or out
- the addition of music, a universal joy

RECREATIONAL AEROBIC DANCE CLASSES: GENERAL PRINCIPLES OF LEADERSHIP

Before you condemn, criticize or abuse, walk a mile in his shoes.

—Ambrose Brazelton

In Maryhelen Vannier's book *Recreation Leadership,* seven principles are cited. I will expand upon these in relation to recreational aerobic dance.

1. **A real leader makes more leaders.** Since recreational aerobic dance routines are choreographed with the non-dancer in mind, motivated individuals can teach others via this activity textbook. Some may joyfully go one step further and make their own routines. The physical educators have been doing this for years. True, but the principle of continuous movement was not employed. Often boredom and a low degree of actual physical exertion resulted. Do not be discouraged, however. Be flexible enough in your thinking to adapt new scientific fitness information and innovative program procedures to your methods and materials. The combination will be pleasingly rewarding.

2. **A true leader gets his or her lead from someone or something greater than himself or herself.** "The leader must be a follower of an idea or ideal that embodies religious concepts and democracy. These guiding stars should chart his course of action, aid him in progressing through troubled waters, and beach him on the shore of accomplishment." Recreational dance aerobics is a joyful, uplifting fitness program. It renews the spirit like no other. When the spirit is renewed, happiness pours out over all.

3. **A real leader has a high degree of expectancy in each group member.** Humans of all ages want to be challenged to their capacities. The gap between potential and accomplishment is lessened through appropriate and effective challenge. The end

result being a higher degree of self-realization, the first Cardinal Principle of Education.

4. **A true leader must support and believe in his group and each member in it.** A good leader learns names early, and recognizes each individual's outstanding qualities and possible limitations. He or she works with the group, not against it, to accomplish the desired goals. An effective leader shows pride in the group's achievements, being very free with encouraging compliments.

5. **The best leader uses the positive approach.** Whereas putdowns cause frustration, feelings of inferiority and futility, the positive approach enhances the self-concept and encourages growth towards self-direction.

6. **The true leader is skilled in working with people and objects.** An effective leader motivates individuals to achieve worthwhile goals such as fun, fitness, fellowship, and fulfillment.

7. **A real leader looks and acts the part of a leader.** The recreational dance aerobics leader should personify holistic fitness. He or she must be a role model, worthy of emulation.

TEACHING SUGGESTIONS

- Discuss the concept of recreational dance aerobics and what the class will involve. Have the students introduce themselves by the end of the second class meeting.
- Cite objectives, expectations and evaluation procedures.
- Refer to information included in this text at various times throughout the course.
- Emphasize safety precautions; have a physical examination if you are over thirty-five or in questionable health, pace yourself and stay within your limits.
- Demonstrate the whole routine or the first major part to music, after introducing the routine and its purpose.
- Teach one step, then do it with the students to music, calling out the cues or major directions ahead of time (ending the cue the beat before the step is to begin).
- Lead the students, seldom facing them. However, be aware of how they are progressing and where they need help. When facing them be sure to use your professional right

and left (you use the left when they are to use the right).

- Review any part that is difficult, emphasizing the timing.
- Repeat steps to the music, keeping the tempo a bit slower until participants pick it up, machine permitting.
- Lessen the number of cues as students improve to avoid detracting from their enjoyment.
- Keep fun and continuous movement your goals, not perfection of steps or body position.
- Determine the number of steps to teach, according to the age of the participants, time available, difficulty of the steps, and the ability and experience of the students.
- Know the dances and music extremely well. Cue cards will help you memorize the steps. Listing major steps on the chalkboard will aid everyone. Be precise and positive.
- Evaluate via written positive and negative comments at midpoint and at the end of the course. These are most helpful to an instructor. Remember, old habits are hard to change and none of us see ourselves as others see us.
- Dance on a wood floor with ample space for the activity, and encourage comfortable clothing and supportive tennis shoes.
- Use the full time, beginning and ending on time.

Scheduling Recreational Dance Aerobics Classes

For secondary/adult levels, classes should be held three times a week on alternating days for at least thirty minutes. Since experience has shown that women can best arrange to take two forty-five minute or one-hour classes per week, it behooves them to jog or participate in another aerobic activity in place of the third session. College students in physical education, recreation, dance or fitness should participate every other day, if possible.

To choreograph a short routine creatively and present it to the class is desirable. This activity will provide practical experience for future leaders. School youngsters need to have the opportunity to engage in this activity as part of a dance or fitness unit. It can provide a "breath of fresh air to the physical education curriculum."

Sample Class Format

1. Warm-up Phase (five to ten minutes). The warm-up con-

sists of stretching exercises for the arms, legs and back. It available, a ballet barre is helpful. Also, do bent-knee sit-ups and push-ups on a mat. Progress to disco moves and line dances.

2. Aerobic Phase (twenty to thirty minutes). Eventually six to eight aerobic dance routines can be performed during this time segment by repeating selected dances, exercising vigorously.

3. Cooldown Phase (five to ten minutes). This time is spent doing one or two cooldown routines, then calf stretches.

Heart Rate Monitoring

Participants should check their heart rate several times during the aerobic phase while walking between routines, to determine if they are getting the desired training effect. If the heart rate does not reach the lower number of the target zone, more exertion is suggested. If the heart rate is above the target zone, the individual is pushing her body too hard for the degree of fitness. A slower pace is indicated.

As for mechanics, preferably, participants should check their heart rate by placing the thumb on the chin and the fingers just off center over the carotid artery of the neck, then be timed for six seconds on the stopwatch of the instructor. At first, the instructor verbally asks for these numbers. Students add a zero to get beats per minute. A visual aid is helpful. After a change of pace, if the heart rate is still out of line, the individual should see a physician before continuing activity.

After the cooldown, monitor the heart rate again. Time the heart rate for fifteen seconds then multiply by four. After a five minute cooldown it should not be higher than one hundred twenty beats per minute, says Dr. Cooper. If higher, the individual should dance at a lower level during future classes until more conditioned.

Calculation of Individual Target Zones

The target heart rate is the heart rate which should be attained when a conditioning effect is desired. Calculated for a sixteen and a forty year-old:

220 - age (sixteen) = 204 maximal heart rate, age adjusted
220 - age (forty) = 180 maximal heart rate, age adjusted

The target zone is between seventy percent and eighty-five percent of the maximal heart rate, plus or minus ten. Above eighty-five percent there is little added benefit from a great deal of extra exercise. This formula has the approval of the American Medical Association.

		Target Zones:
70% X 204 = 143	70% X 180 = 126	143-173 age 16
85% X 204 = 173	80% X 180 = 153	126-153 age 40

Karvonnen's formula takes individual differences into account. Both formulas are accepted; the former represents averages. Calculated for a sixteen and a forty year-old:

220—age = A maximal heart rate, age adjusted
maximal heart rate—resting heart rate = b

```
          .70
  b    X .85 = c
RHR +   c  = d
```

		Target Zones:
180 — 70 RHR = 110	110 X .85 = 94	
110 X .70 = 77	70 + 94 = 164	147-164 age 40
70 + 77 = 147		

		Target Zones:
220 — 80 RHR = 124	124 X .85 = 105	
124 X .70 = 87	80 + 105 = 185	167-185 age 16
80 + 87 = 167		

When figuring training effect, remember it is ± ten beats. If an individual is more than ten beats outside the upper target boundary, there is need for a change of pace.

Just after participants begin the recreational dance aerobics program they should check their resting heart rate in the early morning. At the end of the ten or fifteen week program, check the resting heart rate again. Having gained in physical fitness, it should be lower.

HISTORY OF AEROBIC DANCE

Boring? Never! The history of aerobic dance is exciting! Although aerobic dance has been called fitness fantasia, aerobic fitness, rhythmical aerobics, fitness dancing, jazz-ercise and recreational dance aerobics the commonality is joyful continuous movement for cardiovascular fitness via dance potpourri. The majority of the students now wear supportive tennis shoes, gym shorts, and T-shirts. There are usually no mirrors on the walls. The instructor works with her back to the group. In this way, there is no embarrass-ment, supervision, or implied criticism. Everyone works at a different pace—walking, jogging, or running through the routines. The heart rate is monitored after aerobic routines, so that the amount of exertion is individually safe for each participant.

Aerobic dancing, this innovative physical fitness activity, had its beginnings in 1969, when Jacki Sorensen hosted a television fitness program at the Air Force base in Puerto Rico. Using her knowledge of aerobic exercise obtained from Dr. Ken Cooper's bestseller, *Aerobics*, she put together a remarkably enjoyable course. Women kept asking for more!

Aerobic dancing made its first commercial appearance in 1971. When Jacki's husband, Neil, was transferred to New Jersey, Jacki decided to teach an aerobic dance class to six women in the basement of the South Orange Y.M.C.A. By the time her husband was transferred again in 1972, Jacki was teaching twenty-five classes a week. Aerobic dancing classes replaced the coffee klatch as the favorite morning pastime. Women were beginning to take their bodies serious-ly. Child-bearing was no longer considered a legitimate ex-cuse for being flabby and out of shape.

The President's Council on Physical Fitness and Sports appointed Jacki as a Clinic Staff member in 1972. The Coun-cil has rated aerobic dancing as one of the best overall forms of exercise, right up there with tennis and handball. It strengthens the heart, increases muscle endurance, bolsters muscle power, aids balance and develops body flexibility.

In 1974, Neil Sorensen left his airplane-insurance broker-age to become the chairman of the Aerobic Dancing Corpo-ration. He was the token male in a business otherwise run by one-time housewives. However, now two male instructors are encouraging special programs for men at some centers.

Fun and fitness are addicting! According to Jacki, ninety percent or more of the women return for another session. "When you know what it's like to be physically fit, you never want to quit exercising. You're hooked for life!" Testimonials are numerous from the sixty thousand women involved in twelve-week programs taught by Jacki's one thousand eight hundred contracted instructors. From four main centers in New York, San Diego, Baltimore, and Los Angeles, aerobic dancing has spread to thirty-four states under the guidance and direction of seventy-two regional managers. The far-reaching effects of the aerobic dancing phenomenon have touched Canada, Thailand, Australia and Venezuela.

Yes, the concept of aerobic dancing has snowballed. However, many "straight dance people" look upon this "young upstart" with chagrin. They resent the use of the term dance in such a charleton way. Granted, the aerobic element consists of basic locomotor movements (not foreign to dance). Yes, aerobic dance is a unique concept. Rather than being a traditional type of dance, it is dance potpourri. As variety is the spice of life, aerobic dance offers disco, aerobic folk, aerobic exercise, boogie, snappy jazz and ballet all rolled into one. This winning combination has brought health, physical education, recreation, and dance together in one program. The activity is a sampling of the best from all worlds, with possibilities unlimited. Like the American people, aerobic dance will prosper, not in spite of its unique differences but because of them.

Television coverage has noticeably increased. Commercial sports clubs and recreation departments are trying to meet the demand for more classes. Educators are beginning to recognize its merit. A touring aerobic dance group has been very well received in Y's, colleges, universities and recreation establishments.

Not to be outdone, youngsters are claiming a bit of the fitness spotlight. Some eighty elementary schools in and around Scarborough, Ontario begin the day with twelve minutes of the Health Hustle. Colorado's Aerobic Angels promote fitness by taking part in CAHPERD Fitness Clinics, performing at state conventions and bringing cheer to senior citizens at nursing homes.

However, scattered efforts must be reinforced by a determined new commitment in promoting physical fitness for all, says Carson Conrad, Executive Director of the President's Council on Physical Fitness and Sports. The hard fact is that scores on the national youth fitness test have not improved at all in fifteen years, notes former President Carter.

Obviously, there must be more involvement in viable fitness programs at all grade levels. It's fun! It's worthwhile! Hopefully, we will see a happier, more totally fit America.

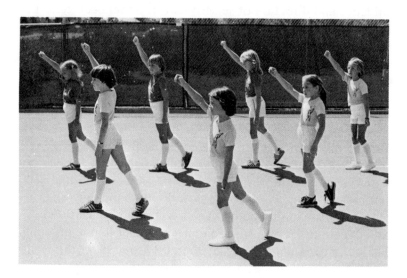

WHY RECREATIONAL DANCE AEROBICS WILL LIVE

"One of the greatest problems with exercise is the boredom experienced by the average person. Aerobics makes exercise more pleasurable, and therefore, people will stay with the program longer," states N.R. Van Dinter, Associate Professor at the University of Northern Colorado. Besides banishing the boring, this joyful terpsichorean activity pleases the eye, nurtures the intellect, and inspires the soul. It is based on the sound principles of recreation, which is people-oriented.

Where is man without good health? Fitness and health are of the utmost importance. Through laboratory tests, it has been shown that aerobic dancing offers long-term health rewards. In a 1971 study, one hundred fifty women at Immaculata College in Pennsylvania took Dr. Cooper's twelve minute running test. Half of the group was designated as a control group and continued their normal activities. The other half was enrolled in a four-times-a-week, twelve-week aerobic dance program.

At the conclusion of the twelve weeks, both groups were tested again. Using Dr. Cooper's chart, pre-program tests of the dance group showed sixty-one percent in the Very Poor and Poor categories, with five percent in the Good category. None scored Excellent. In contrast, post-program tests showed twenty-five percent had moved into the Good category and three percent had advanced to Excellent. In addition, some participants showed a loss of as much as four inches in hip measurements and ten pounds in weight. The control group showed little change, with eight percent in the Good category initially, then ten percent after twelve weeks.

Research by Weber showed the oxygen consumption was twenty-nine milliliters per kilogram per minute for a thirty-minute work period. He concluded that both the intensity and duration of exercise was sufficient to elicit a training effect. Foster confirmed Weber's findings at the University of Texas in 1973. The oxygen consumption represented a physiological disturbance comparable to running a twelve-minute mile pace.

Based on sound physiological principles, aerobic dancing has and will withstand the weathering of time....the thoughtful man built his house on the rock. The rains came down, the floods rose, the winds beat upon that house, but it never collapsed, for it was based on the rock. The foolish man built his house on the sand. The rains came down....and the wreck of it was complete.

—Matthew 8:24

In a later study in 1974, Dr. Herb Weber of East Stroudsburg State College in Pennsylvania measured energy expenditure for moderate intensity aerobic dancing sessions as comparable to ice skating at nine miles per hour, walking at three and one-half miles per hour, or bicycling at ten miles per hour. For high-intensity sessions, he found that the energy expenditure was equivalent to a half hour of vigorous basketball, cycling at thirteen miles per hour, running at five and one-half miles per hour, and swimming at fifty-five yards per minute. In terms of calories, aerobic dancing for forty-five minutes at the walking level will burn approximately one hundred seventy kilocalories, two hundred eighty kilocalories at the jogging level, and four hundred kilocalories at the running level.

More recent studies were conducted by Veronica Igbanugo and Dr. Bernard Gutin at Teachers College of Columbia University. The women utilized 3.96 kilocalories per minute for the low-intensity routine, 6.28 kilocalories per minute for the medium-intensity routine and 7.75 kilocalories per minute for the high-intensity routine. The men utilized 4.17 kilocalories per minute for the low-intensity routine, 6.86 kilocalories per minute for the medium and 9.44 kilocalories per minute at the high-intensity level.

The energy expenditure for the low intensity routine was metabolically similar to walking, that of medium-intensity to playing tennis, and that of high-intensity to playing hockey. Mean heart rates for women were one hundred fourteen, one hundred forty-five, and one hundred fifty-six beats per minute and one hundred six, one hundred twenty-nine, and one hundred forty-one for men.

Igbanugo and Dr. Gutin concluded that the medium and high-intensity dance levels provide adequate stress to influence the efficiency of the cardiovascular system. The low-intensity level can provide adequate exercise for the early stages of a program for recently bedridden patients or patients recovering from heart attacks, agrees cardiologist John L. Boyer of San Diego.

Results of recent laboratory research by Lenore R. Zohman, M.D., and Albert A. Kattus, M.D., internationally acclaimed exercise cardiologists, showed among other things that the relationship of heart rates and oxygen consumption while carrying out fitness dancing was the same as when on the treadmill. That is, the points measured as low, middle, and high level dancing fell right on the heart rate oxygen consumption line determined from the mill. This made possible comparable data, (including energy cost values), thus simplifying techniques.

Music sets the pace for dancing, not the instructor. The three fitness levels of participation enable each person to move at his or her own energy level, yet enjoy the company of others. Since basic locomotor movements are used, people who don't know how to dance still fit right in. Everyone achieves. The self concept is enhanced, and individuals feel good about themselves.

Recreational dance aerobics is a social activity. Being gregarious by nature, most people enjoy people. According to psychologist Jonathan Friedman, "Crowding tends to intensify our reactions to a particular sensation." In this case, it's the joy of moving in a group to stimulating music. Without competition, comradery is enhanced.

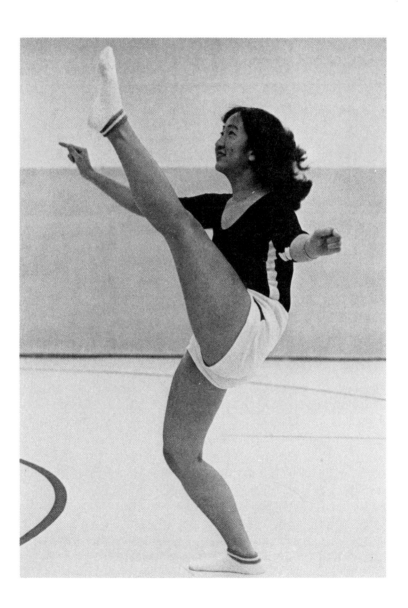

There is a destiny which makes us brothers—none goes his way alone. All that we send into the lives of others comes back into our own.

—Markham the Poet

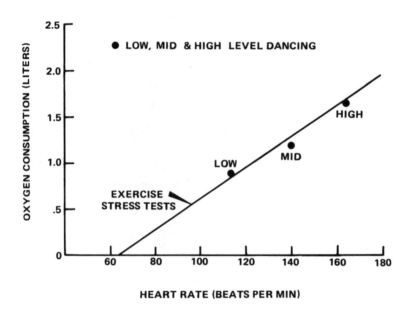

Source: *The Cardiologists' Guide to Fitness and Health Through Exercise*. Copyright © 1979 by Lenore R. Zohman, M.D., Albert A. Kattus, M.D., and Donald G. Softness, Simon and Schuster, New York. Reprinted by permission of the author and publisher.

Part Three
Original Dance
Aerobics Routines

No art provided primitive man with as diversified and complex a vehicle of expression as the dance, for he developed it from the simple prancing and preening of the animals, danced out of sheer physical exuberance, courtship, ritual and need to communicate.

—Walter Terry

The following section of this text contains fifteen original dance aerobic routines, choreographed specifically for inclusion in the warm-up, aerobic, or cooldown phase of the recreational dance aerobics fitness program. Both the steps and the routines build progressively so that peak exertion takes place during the aerobic phase. After twenty minutes within the target zone, the tapering off period begins.

In order to allow for individual differences, especially in age and degree of fitness, three levels of participation are possible. Move from one level into another as needed.

Walking Level

1. Walk instead of jogging to the music.

2. Omit hops, jumps, slides, and polkas.

3. Keep arm movements to a minimum.

Jogging Level

1. Do the routines, more or less like the leader.

2. Include the hops, jumps, slides and polkas.

3. Dance at a moderately high level of exertion.

Running Level

1. Raise the knees high on the jogs, while covering as much distance as possible, considering the formation.

2. Reach, swing, or move the arms at a high energy level.

3. Execute all kicks and jumps with vigor and elevation.

Participants should have a complete physical examination before beginning any physically active training program.

Warm-Up Phase

Stretching should begin the warm-up phase. These exercises are to be done slowly and progressively. Additional time spent warming-up will prevent tendon and musculoskeletal problems. Specifically, hold each stretch position for about thirty seconds without straining. *Never bob or bounce*! The rationale is that a protective sensor system in each muscle automatically reacts to a sudden stretch; a reflex action occurs inhibiting elongation. This results in tightening. "Tightness limits the enjoyment of movement and the development of personal potential," says Bobby Anderson. Do not hold your breath. Relax. Stretch easily, breathe slowly and rhythmically.

Disco rhythms challenge like no other. Basic locomotor movements done to catchy disco tunes become great fun! Success is immediate. With joy, the heart rate increases progressively.

"The disco beat is hypnotic. I'll dance till the day I die," exclaims Disco Sally, a retired lawyer who at age seventy-seven, dances every night at New York's Studio 54.

"The hustle reminds me of an encounter group with rhythm," says Erma Bombeck. "Take disco...please."

ROUTINE NUMBER 1: Stretching

MUSIC: "Tracy's Theme" and "Climb Every Mountain" or other slow music.

TIME: 5:16 Minutes

DIRECTIONS: Hold all stretches twenty to thirty seconds. Do not bounce or bob. Repeat several times on both sides where possible. (Photos L to R).

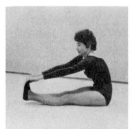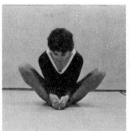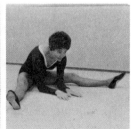

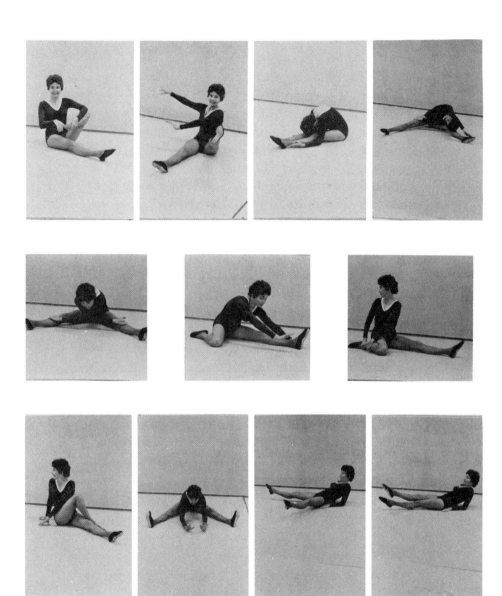

SITTING POSITION:

1. Pull on the toes while legs are extended and together, so that the heels come off the floor.
2. Lean forward with soles of the feet together and the hands over the toes.
3. Put forearms down or at least toward the floor while

the legs are in straddle position with toes pointed.

4. Bring the lower leg toward the chest.

5. Extend the held leg diagonally out to the side, arms extending toward the opposite side.

6. Bring the nose down to the knees, with legs together and forward, hands along the lower legs.

7. Bring the opposite arm up and over to touch the toes, while in straddle position. The other arm is crossed at the waist holding the opposite thigh. Lower the torso sideways, placing the ear down toward the knee.

8. Bring the upper arm across to the remaining thigh, lean forward.

9. Flex the feet in hurdle position, reach toward the forward foot.

10. Lean forward as you move the hands to the opposite ankle in a sweeping motion. Twist the upper back toward the bent leg. Repeat. Lean, then go up on R knee—R hand also supporting.

11. Flex one leg and place it on the floor beside the outside of the opposite knee. Twist away from the legs and hold.

12. Lean forward and stretch with legs straight and feet flexed.

13. Straddle, then cross the ankles, keeping the legs as close to the floor as possible, while supporting your weight on the forearms.

14. Straddle and cross with the other leg on top.

15. V sit by bringing the legs diagonally forward and parallel to the arms.

16. Elevate the legs in the V as you bring the arms horizontally out to the sides.

17. Hold where it hurts when going down in position for sit-ups, relax in supine position, then sit up.

18. Swing one leg horizontally from the side crossing in front while the other leg is flexed, arms moving in opposition.

19. Swing the same leg back out to the side, arms swing to the opposite side.

20. Lift the top leg up as you support yourself sideways on one forearm and hand.

21. Lower the top leg as the lower leg comes to meet it.

22. Separate the legs vertically, then bring them to rest on the floor.

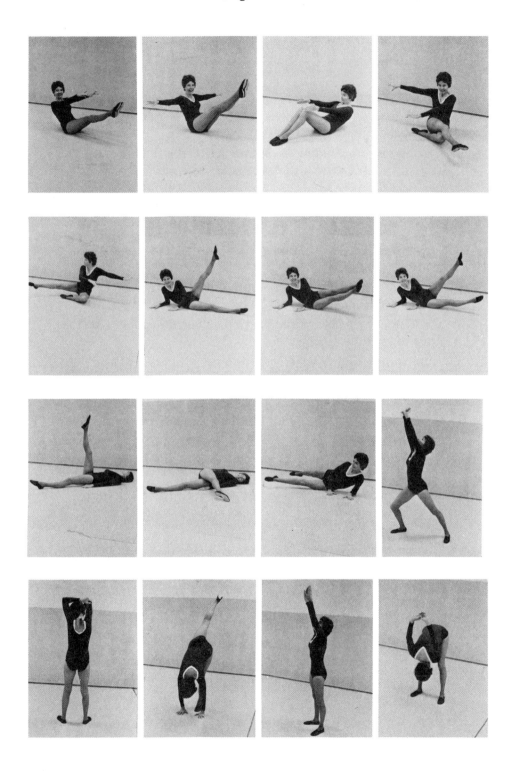

SUPINE POSITION:

23. Execute leg overs by bringing one leg up to a vertical position.
24. Bring the extended leg down to touch the floor directly across from the hip. Bring it to a vertical position again, then down beside the other leg.
25. Scissor the legs holding them parallel to the floor, while resting on one hip supported by one forearm and hand.

STANDING POSITION:

26. Lunge and stretch the palms toward the ceiling.
27. Flex one arm above the head (hand down the back) and lower that hand by elbow pressure from the opposite side.
28. Place the hands flat on the floor as you lift one leg extended vertically in back.
29. Cross the wrists placing the palms together, extending the arms toward the ceiling.
30. Holding one thumb, lean forward letting the arms extend vertically.

ALL FOURS POSITION:

31. Walk forward on the hands stopping directly under the shoulders, elevating the feet.
32. Flex the arms touching the chin or chest on the floor (depending how lucky you are), then extend.
33. Lift one leg horizontally to the side (eye focus on the moving leg), swing the leg backward horizontally past the midline.
34. Having swung the leg back, swing to starting position. Increase in speed. Add the arm swing (same side as leg), swinging away from the leg horizontally, then horizontally crossing.

SUPINE POSITION:

35. Push-up bridge or back bend position with the hands directly under the shoulders, fingers pointing toward shoulders, getting a greater stretch than with sit-ups.

STANDING POSITION:

36. Bring the leg to the chest into flexed position, hands on lower leg.

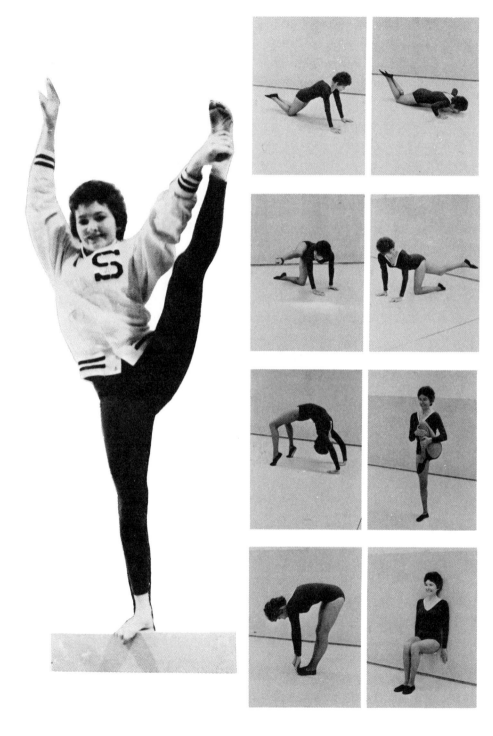

37. Lean forward and pull on the toes.

38. Wall sit, making a ninety-degree angle at the knees, holding this position as long as possible.

Touch Dancin' by Murtour Battle ("Mr. B")

Use current disco music. Repeat each step several times. R means right, L means left.

Photos (L to R)	Steps
1,2	1. Touch R, step R, touch L, step L, repeat touching in back.
3,4	2. Step side R, close L, step side R, kick L (clap), step side L, close R, step side L, kick R (clap).
	3. Touch R foot to the side, step R beside L, touch L foot out to the side, step L beside R.
7,8,9	4. Pelvic Moves (legs flexed). Improvise.
10	5. R heel, step R, L heel, step L.
10,11	6. Step L, brush R foot forward, brush R foot back (flexed) crossing over L, brush R forward, step R, tap L foot twice behind R (you can tap L hand on the floor twice).
12	7. Step R into a wide stride position (knees flexed), and pull bent arms back twice (pelvis forward twice), close L beside R (still flexed) pull arms back twice (pelvis forward twice), step L with L (pulling arms back twice), close R beside L pulling arms back twice.
13,14	8. Do shoulder isolations by lifting the R shoulder then the L shoulder.
15,16	9. Do a one quarter turn, step L forward, brush R forward and step on it, touch L beside R as you face ninety degrees to the L, step back L, step back R facing front, touch L.
21-29	10. Robot moves.

Monorail Line Dance to "Heaven Knows" or similar music. Jump front (hold), jump back (hold), scoot R, L (quick steps forward), scoot R, L. Jump feet apart, jump feet together. R

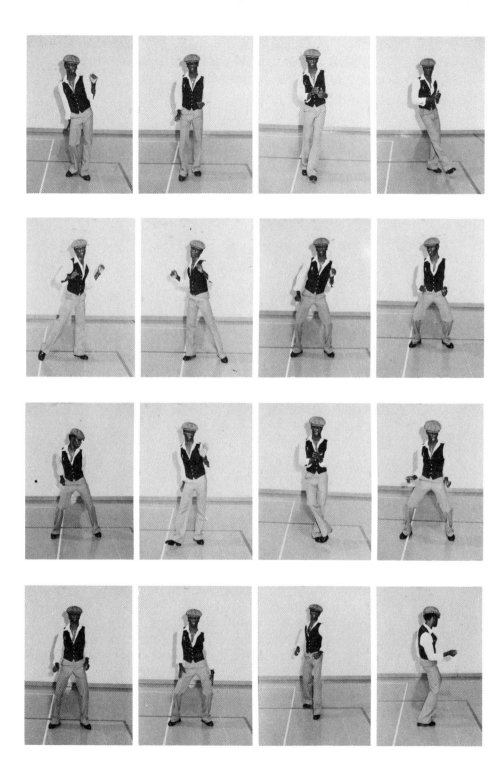

heel front, step R. L heel front, step L. Stiff legged low
march R, L. Step forward on R and pivot slowly to the L
ninety degrees. Repeat until music ends.

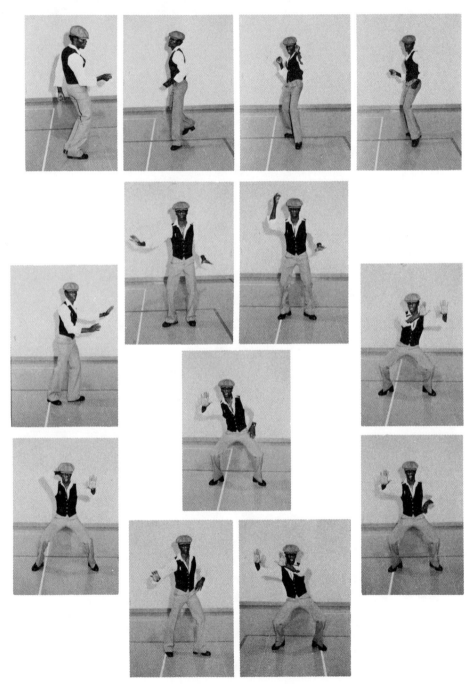

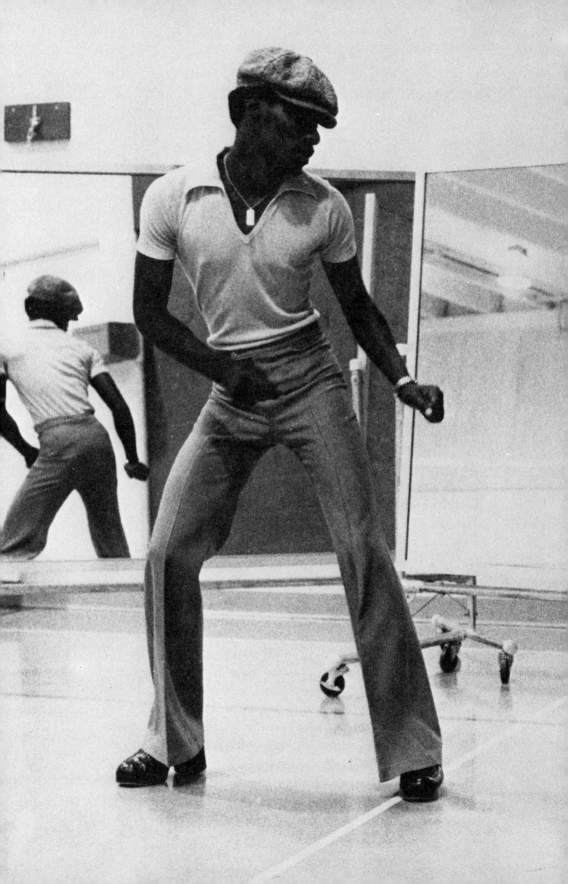

ROUTINE NUMBER 2: Chocolate Hustle Line Dance

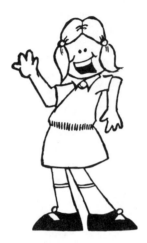

MUSIC: "Makin It," "Center of My Heart," "YMCA," or
       "Funkytown."

TIME: 3:30 Minutes

BASIC ACTION INCLUDES: Suzi Q, Walks, Rock, Grape-
       vine. Later, hop it all, omitting Suzie Q.

STARTING FORMATION: Stand in alternate columns fac-
       ing front.

Step Number 1

Counts

16   a.   Grapevine—do four (R L R L). Step R, cross L,
            step R to the R, kick L to the L (clap). Repeat
            L etc.

8   b.   Suzi Q—do two sets (RL). With feet together,
           move toes R, then move heels R, move toes R,
           low kick L to the L. When learning, just do
           four R then L without the kick. Add Suzi Q
           later.

4   c.   Walk—do four (moving backward R L R),
           bring bent L leg up (lean back).

4   d.   Rock—do three (forward, back, forward), pivot
           ninety degrees L on L with R leg bent.

     Note: If you are using this basic line dance variation
           or others with children or seniors (all love it),
           skip the pivot temporarily. Just pause and keep

CHOCOLATE HUSTLE

Grapevine Right

Suzie-Q

Walks

Rock

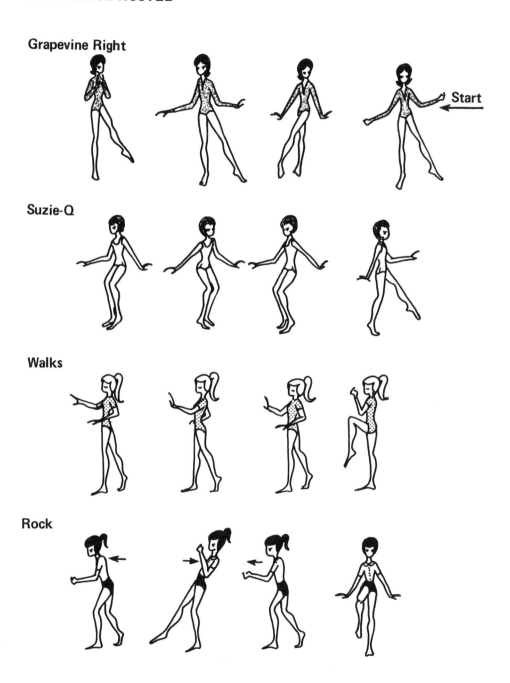

facing front until the steps are mastered. After this early success experience, when participants are comfortable with it, add the pivot. Jog the grapevine steps to make it more aerobic on the second or third lesson. Do at least one square at the walk pace so it builds cardiovascularly.

ROUTINE NUMBER 3: Rockin' Combo

MUSIC: "I Remember Yesterday," Donna Summer.

TIME: 3:38 Minutes

BASIC ACTION INCLUDES: Touch Close, Walks, Basic Hustle, Three Step Turns, Jumps, Twists, Grapevine, Jabs, Boogie, Rock, Pennsylvania Hustle, Touches.

STARTING FORMATION: Standing in alternate columns facing front, feet apart, arms low and diagonal, eyes down.

NOTE: First teach the Bus Stop in a continuous square to slow music such as: "Stayin' Alive," "Jive Talkin'," "Heaven Knows," or "More Than a Woman." About the third lesson, teach the Pennsylvania Hustle, then on the fifth or sixth lesson teach the Rollercoaster. Keep reviewing them. Finally, do the Hot Disco Combo.

Introductory Poses

Counts

1	a.	arms up (snap on each of the eight counts)
2		R arm horizontally to the R, L arm down, eyes R
3		R arm down, L up (bend arms when changing positions)
4		R arm up, L arm down
5		R arm horizontally to the R, L arm up, eyes R
6		Close L foot beside R, slap thighs
7		arms straight up
8		arms down, pause backward full arm circle crossing the arms above the head, ending in a low diagonal (fingers together). If using the record, repeat the same movements (eight counts)

ROCKIN' COMBO

**Instruction
Coordinator**

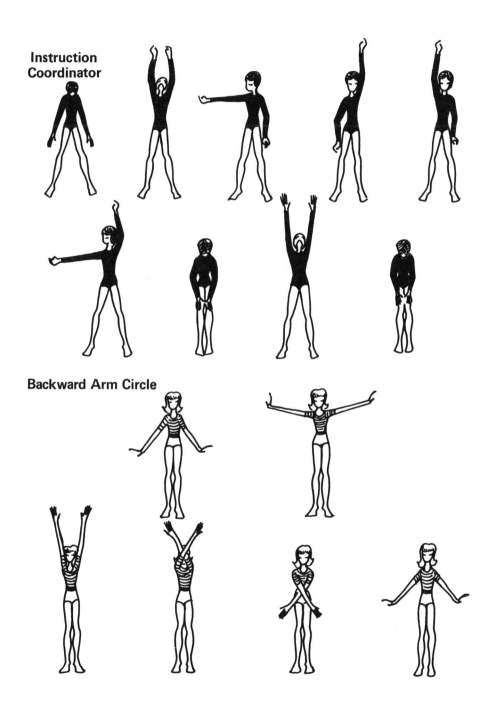

Backward Arm Circle

16   b.   Touch close—do two (R to the side, R close beside L), do two (L side, L close), do two (R front, R close), do two (L front, L close).

8   c.   Walk—do three forward (R L R touch L beside R, clap or snap), do three backward (L R L touch R, clap).

Step Number 1: Bus Stop

8   a.   Hustle—touch with the R. Do two front, two back, one front one back (not shown), one side, low kick forward as pivot ninety degrees L.

8   b.   Walks—do three backward (R L R touch L, clap or snap). Do three forward (L R L touch R, clap).

8   c.   Three Step Turns—do two (step R to the side, step one hundred eighty degrees onto L, step R one hundred eighty degrees, touch L (clap). Arms are curved and horizontal. Repeat to the L.

8   d.   Straight kicks—do two straight kicks (R   L), half bends (flex legs twice).
backward then forward twice as you flex or bend, then straighten the legs twice.

128   Repeat step number 1 four more times, the last time while facing front.

Large Break

16   a.   Forearm Circle—walk diagonally R circling forearms (R L R touch L, circle or clap as touch). Walk backward (L R L touch R). Repeat walks moving diagonally L then repeat walks backward.

4   b.   Fever Touches—touch R foot to the side (point R index finger high diagonally R, cross R foot behind L (pointing R index finger low diagonally L). Repeat.

4   c.   Heel Clicks—after a step R, close L (place thumbs in arm pits. Do two heel clicks (turn toes in, hit heels and flap elbows).

Touch Close

Start

Front Close

Start

Walks

Clap

Start

Start

Clap

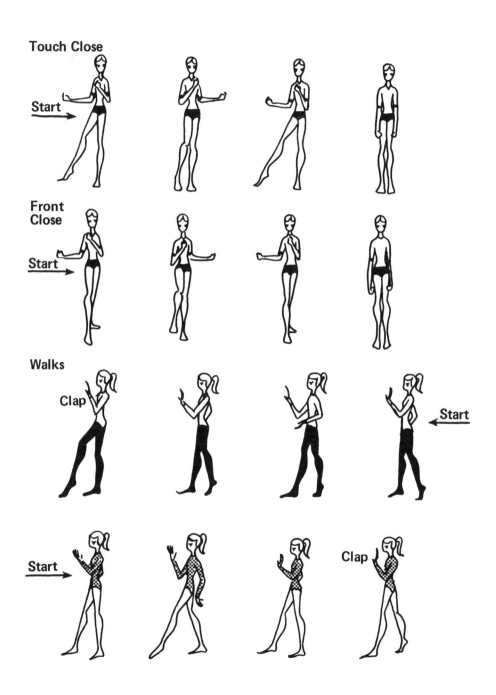

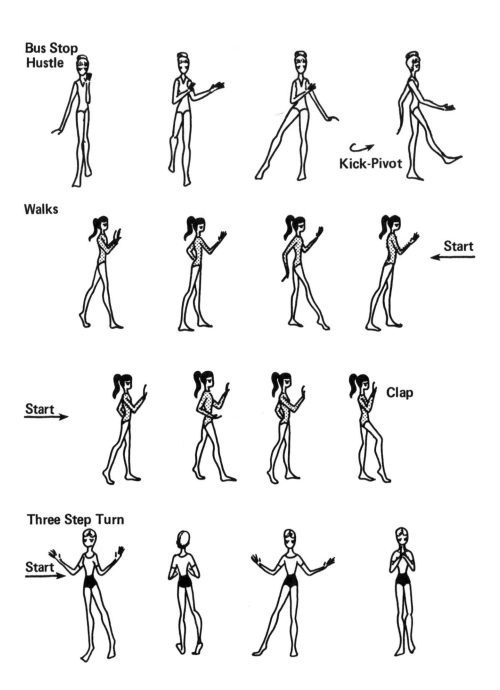

Bus Stop Hustle

Kick-Pivot

Walks

Start

Start

Clap

Three Step Turn

Start

Jump, Twist

Forearm Circle

Walk Back

Fever Touches

Heel Clicks

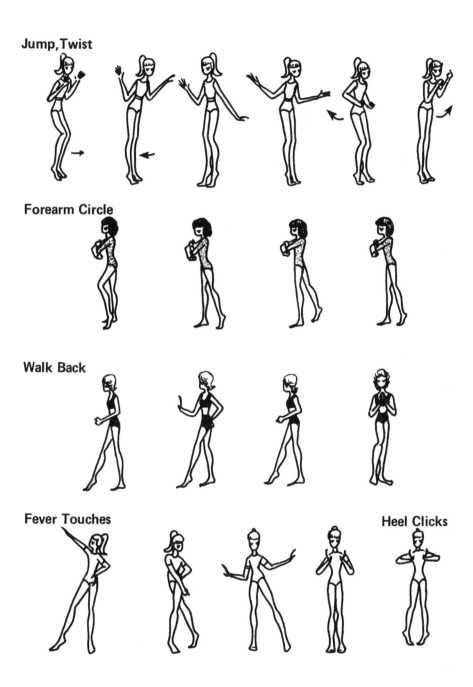

Step Number 2: Rollercoaster (begins on "I saw your love light.....").

8   a.   Grapevine—do two (step side R, cross L over R, step R, kick L to the L). Repeat beginning L.

4   b.   Jab—jump onto R with L heel forward (toes up). Change or switch feet so R heel is forward, change so L heel is forward. Flex and cross L leg in front of R.

2   c.   Boogie—step on L (R leg bent knee out) R arm straight down, and L bent. Switch arm position so L is straight and R is bent (R knee in).

2   Step on R foot (L leg bent with knee turned in). R arm is straight with L bent. Switch arms position turning L knee out.

4   d.   Rock—shift weight onto back foot, step forward onto L, shifting the weight forward, shift weight backward, pivot on L foot ninety degrees to the L.

140   Repeat step number 2 seven more times making two squares moving counterclockwise.

Small Break (When you face front).

8   a.   Suzi Q—move toes R, heels R, toes R, heels R. Repeat L.

Step Number 3: Pennsylvania Hustle

5   a.   With L foot: touch side, touch together, touch side, touch side, close.

5   b.   With R foot: touch front, touch back, touch front, touch back, step.

6   c.   With L foot: touch L over R, touch side, touch L over R, touch side, step L over R pivot ninety degrees to the R, ending with feet together.

48   Repeat three more times ending the routine as you face front.

**Roller Coaster
Grapevine**

Jab

Boogie

Rock

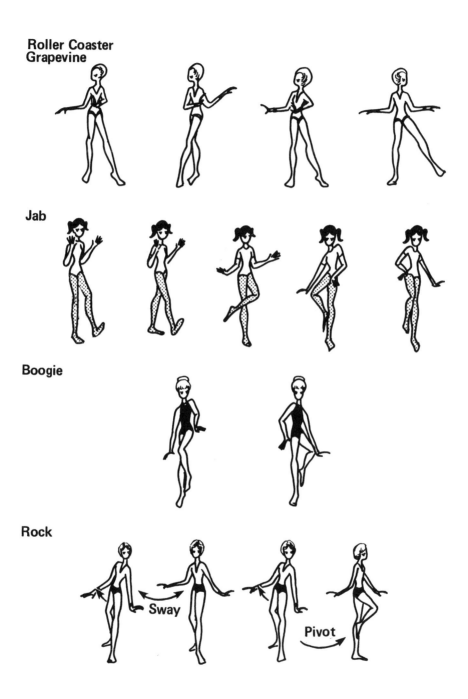

Sway

Pivot

Suzie-Q

Pennsylvania Hustle

Touch Front,Back

Cross touches

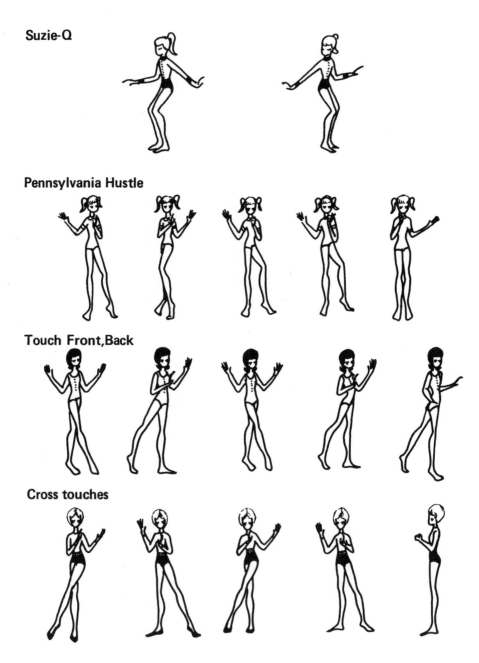

AEROBIC PHASE

The aerobic phase consists of at least twenty minutes of fast locomotor movements while keeping the heart rate within the individual's target zone. A conditioning effect will occur—the desired result of any training program.

Testimonials: Recreational aerobic dance is:

- a "free spirit" type of aerobic movement.
- a lot of fun without realizing you're getting that much exercise.
- gives me a boost after a long day.
- a super good way to have fun and shape up.
- a great form of exercise without the unpleasantness.
- fun and interesting due to the variety of music and steps.
- a great way to loosen up and still have fun.
- great, even though I can't always keep up.
- a lot of fun—highest recommendations to everyone.
- a fun and motivating way to keep fit—delightful music.
- a good way to relieve daily job pressures.
- just what I was looking for—great energy afterwards.
- helping me to lose weight, so I feel much better.
- just great! I will take it again.

ROUTINE NUMBER 4: Dance Variety

MUSIC: "A Night at the Opera"

TIME: 2:57 Minutes

BASIC ACTION INCLUDES: Straight Kicks, Circle Boogie, Kick Ball Change, Suzi Q, Highland I and II, PE Slides, Squat Extensions, Back Boogie, Shorty George, Side Boogie.

STARTING FORMATION: Alternate columns facing instructor.

Step Number 1

Counts

8   a.   Wait eight counts

24   b.   Straight Kicks—do three sets. Kick L R L (arms are flexed and horizontal, snap at neck area as you kick). Kick R (snap) ball (step back onto ball of R foot) change (step on L). Bring the arms down and back on the ball change for more challenge. Instead of straight kicks, as you become more skilled, you may want to circle boogie. Just circle the foot with a low kick (front and out to the side) lifting the hip of the action leg.

Large Break

16   a.   Sunshine Snaps—do four arm circles after stepping R to the R. Begin with a full circle with L arm across body snapping four times. Repeat with the R etc. moving the arm from low to high and across the body.

8   b.   Suzi Q—do four R then four L (move toes R. Then heels R, toes R, heels R, then repeat L).

Step Number 2

8   a.   Highland I—do two (hop touch R foot to the side, hop and bend the leg bringing the foot behind the lower L leg, hop and touch R to the side, hop and flex leg crossing leg in front). The L arm is curved overhead while the R hand is on the hip. On the L side (footwork), the R arm is overhead and L is on the hip. Learn leg movements, then arms.

DANCE VARIETY

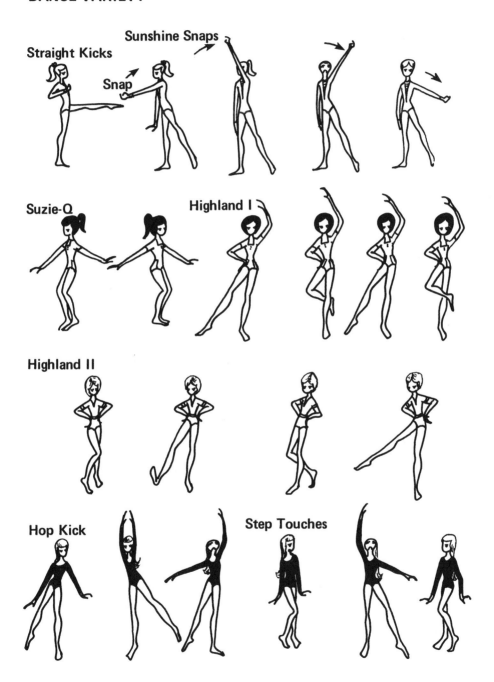

Straight Kicks

Sunshine Snaps

Snap

Suzie-Q

Highland I

Highland II

Hop Kick

Step Touches

8	b.	Skip—do four moving backward with knees out beginning L, then four forward beginning L.
16		Repeat Highland I

Step Number 3

16	a.	Slide and Kick (not shown)—do four sets. Slide to the R three times and kick L foot L. Repeat L, etc.
16	b.	Highland II—With R foot: toe touch (knee in) heel, toe touch behind, kick to the side. Repeat all with L foot, then R, then L. Hands are on the hips.

Large Break

4	a.	Hop, Kick—do two hops on L holding R leg out to the R side (arms out to sides). Do two hops on R with L leg out to the L side (circle and open both arms overhead).
8	b.	Step Digs—do two (step L onto L) (circle L arm across body R to L), dig R twice beside L. Step R dig L twice (circle R arm across body from low L to R above head).
8	c.	Body Bend (not shown)—do one after moving curved arms from low in front overhead opening to the sides, bend forward at the waist sweep hands over toes, open arms again overhead then out to the sides and down.
8	d.	Straight Kicks—do two straight kicks (R L) half bends (flex legs twice).

Step Number 4: Boogie

8	a.	Back Boogie—do four (step back R, feet apart L toes up. Snap and swing R hand across body L to R. Step back L, feet apart R toes up. Snap and swing R hand across body R to L. Repeat R then L.
8	b.	Shorty George—do six (two slow then four fast). Step forward onto R (L leg bent and R arm straight down, L flexed). Step onto L (R leg bent). Repeat R L R L.
16	c.	Side Boogie—step R with R (lift L hip). Touch L beside R, step R (lift hip) touch L beside R.

Back Boogie

Shortie Georgie Boogie

Side Boogie

Aerobic Hop

Start

Squat

Ending

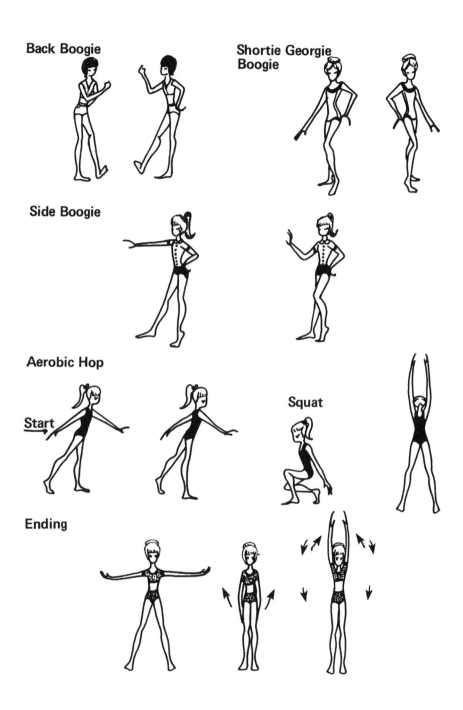

The R arm is horizontally out to the R while the L is on the hip. Repeat L, R, L–totally four sets.

64	Repeat step number 4, Boogie, (twice).

Small Break

16	Suzi Q–do four R, four L, four R, four L. (move toes R, heels R, toes R, heels R).
32	Repeat step number 2, Highland I
32	Repeat step number 3, Slide and Kick, Highland II.

Step Number 5

12	a.	Hop, Kick–hop two times on L holding R leg out to the R sides (arms out). Do two hops on R with L leg out to the L side (circle arms opening overhead). Repeat twice.
16	b.	Back Kicks–run in place L, R, L kicking R leg back hop L. Arms swing parallel to each other and side to side, legs extending backward. Repeat R, L, R–totally four sets.
4	c.	Turn to face center of the circle which you will form. Squat down, extend arms upward jumping to feet-apart position.

Step Number 6

24	a.	PE Slides–do twelve moving counterclockwise.
8	b.	Squat, extend arms upward jumping to feet apart position, jump extending arms out to the sides, jump feet together, arms coming down to the sides. Wave hands with fingers together, up like a Jumping Jack and overhead, then down to the sides.

ROUTINE NUMBER 5: Navy Special

MUSIC: "In the Navy"

TIME: 3:35 Minutes

BASIC ACTION INCLUDES: Aerobic Jumps, PE slides, Polka, Four Count Jumping Jacks, Lunges, Marching, Knee Hook, Hitch Kick, Sunshine Two Step, Horizontal Pulls, Grapevine, Jab and Jogs.

STARTING FORMATION: Several large single circles. Begin after one introductory note.

INTRODUCTION: Aerobic Jumps—do four vertical jumps (clap on the downbeat and pull elbows backward as you land).

Step Number 1

Counts

16   a.   PE Slides—do eight R, eight L (slide to the side pulling flexed arms back on the first slide, and bring them forward on the second, etc., hands in fist position.

16   b.   Polka—do four into center of circle, do four out of circle. Begin R (hop L step R close L step R). Turn R on the fourth one into the center. Turn R on the fourth one coming out of the center of the circle. For less exercise, do two steps.

Step Number 2

4   a.   Four Count Jumping Jacks—do one by jumping to side stride position or feet apart (arms out to sides or second position), jump feet together (hands clap above head), jump to feet apart (arms out to sides), jump feet together (arms down).

4   Jump to small lunge L (R arm low and to the L across body, look L), jump feet together (arms down at sides), jump to small lunge R (L arm low and to the R across body), jump feet together (arms down at sides).

8   Repeat Jumping Jacks and Lunges.

16   b.   March six beginning L and moving clockwise, then turn (to the rear march) i.e., put L foot forward, pivot R (hands on hips for the turn), counts seven, eight. Repeat moving counter-clockwise.

32   Repeat step number 2, Four Count Jumping Jacks.

Step Number 3

16   a.   March to the words "In the Navy," do four

(L R L R) into center of circle, knee hook (jump onto L bringing flexed R leg up) step R, hitch kick (jump onto L as you kick straight R leg forward). Repeat marches moving backward, knee hook, hitch kick.

16   b.   Sunshine Two Step—two step moving to the L beginning L (thumbs under armpits, elbows up), back step R (arms up), step L in place. Repeat R, L, R.

32   Repeat step number 3.

Small Break

8   Aerobic Jumps—do four facing front.

8   Aerobic Jumps—do four turning clockwise in own square.

64   Repeat step number 2, Jumping Jacks (twice).

64   Repeat step number 3, March In (twice).

Large Break

8   Aerobic Jumps—do facing front.

8   Aerobic Jumps—do four turning clockwise in own square

8   Aerobic Jumps—do four facing front. Some must turn.

Step Number 4

8   a.   Horizontal Pulls—do three (R L R slower). Feet apart, pull arms horizontally from side to side keeping them parallel (lean forward, lead with shoulder).

8   b.   Sailor—step L, R jump onto L, R toes up to side (flex arms twice, fist position, elbows out, motion like washing clothes on a board). Repeat beginning R, L, then R.

16   c.   Repeat Horizontal Pulls (L R L slower). Repeat Sailor Step beginning R.

Step Number 5: Rollercoaster

8   a.   Grapevine—do two (step side R, cross L over R, step R, kick L to the L. Repeat beginning L).

4   b.   Jab—jump onto R with L heel forward (toes up). Change or switch feet so R heel is forward,

NAVY SPECIAL

Aerobic Jump   **P.E. Slides**

Polka

Jumping Jacks

Lunge

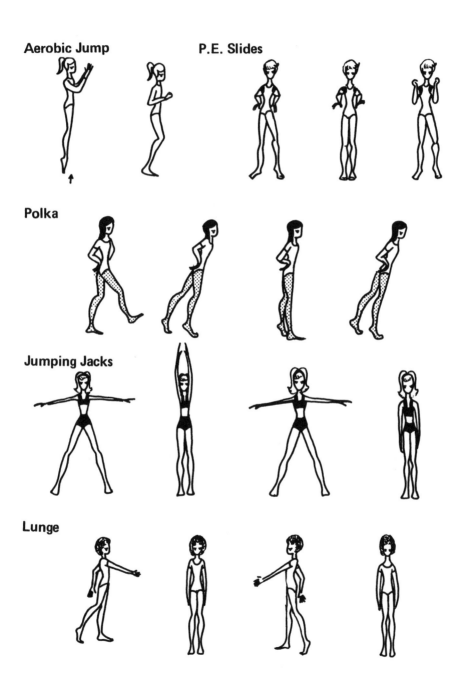

March

Knee Hook
Hitch Kick

Sunshine Two-Step

Aerobic Jumps Square

Horizontal Pulls

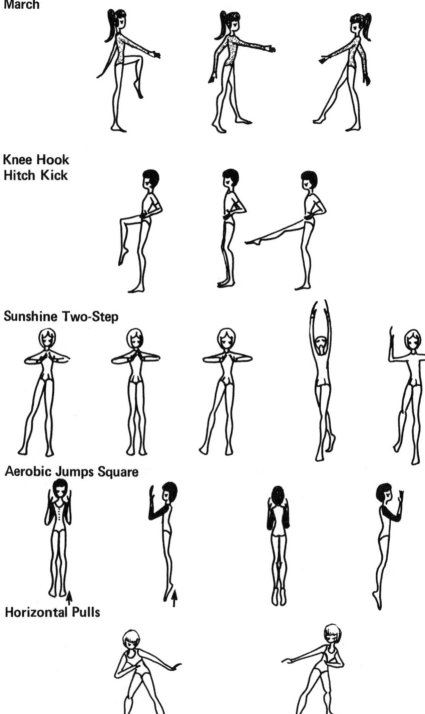

Sailor

Jog

Ending

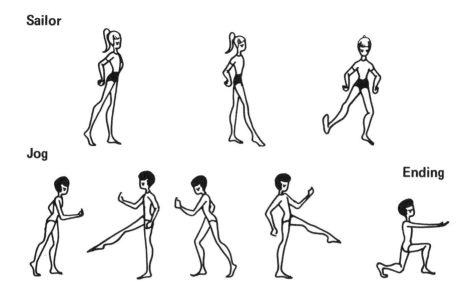

		change so L heel is forward. Flex and cross L leg in front of R.
2	c.	Boogie—step on L (R leg bent with knee out) R arm straight down, and L bent. Switch arm position so L is straight and R is bent (R knee in).
2		Step on R foot (L leg bent with knee turned in). R arm is straight with L bent. Switch arm positions, turning L knee out.
16	d.	Grapevine L, Grapevine R, jab beginning L as above and Boogie.

Small Break

8	Jog L (L R L kick R back and turn to the R). Jog R (R L R kick L back and turn to the L), some turn L to march into center.
32	Repeat step number 3 entirely.

Ending

16	Repeat step number 3 a, b. Sunshine Two Step—do one L, one R except go down on the L knee extending arms forward then stand, hands going onto hips to end.

ROUTINE NUMBER 6: Aerobic Jog

MUSIC: "I Feel Love" by Donna Summer

TIME: 4:00 Minutes

BASIC ACTION INCLUDES: Jogs, Jogs and Kick, Aerobic Jumps, Jumping Jack and Lunge, Polka, Aerobic Taps, PE Slides.

STARTING FORMATION: Alternate lines facing teacher. Wait eight counts.

Step Number 1

Counts

8	a.	Jogs—do eight facing front beginning R.
16	b.	Jog and Kick—jog three (R L R) and kick L low to the L. Do four sets total.
8	c.	Aerobic Jumps—do four in a square moving clockwise, doing the first one facing front.
72		Repeat b and c three more times.

Large Break

16	a.	Jumping Jack and Lunge or four Jumping Jacks—jump feet apart (arms horizontally out to the sides), jump feet together (arms clap overhead), jump feet apart (arms horizontally out to the sides), jump feet together (arms down to sides). Lunge L with body facing L (eyes and R arm low to the L), jump feet together (arms down at sides) lunge R with body facing R (eyes and L arm to R), jump feet together (arms down at sides). Repeat Jumping Jack and Lunge.

Step Number 2

32	a.	Jog—do sixteen jogs moving in a large circle counterclockwise. Repeat doing sixteen jogs clockwise.

Step Number 3

16	a.	Polka—do four moving into the center of the circle, turning R on the fourth one. Do four moving outward, turning R on the fourth one to face center again. Learn as two steps first.
16	b.	Aerobic Taps—do eight. Hop and tap R foot

AEROBIC JOG

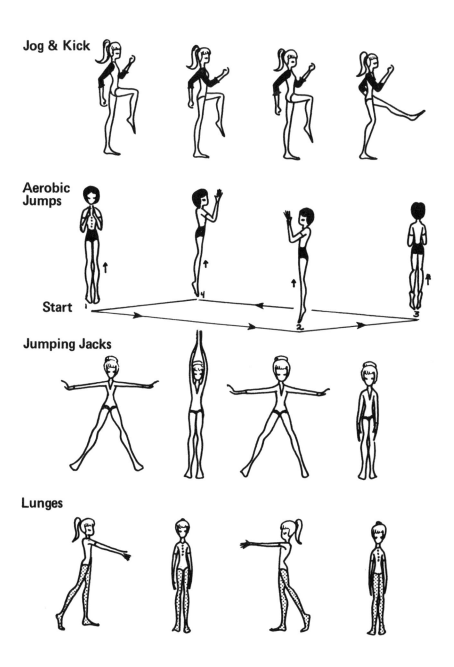

Jog & Kick

Aerobic
Jumps

Start

Jumping Jacks

Lunges

with L hand, hop and touch R foot out to the R side, hop and tap R foot which is bent crossing behind L with L hand, hop and touch R foot out to R side. Repeat R foot taps. Repeat tapping the L foot with R hand, turning a full turn R staying in one spot.

Step Number 4

24   a.   PE Slides—slide eight R or chasse to the R pulling bent arms back fist position, slide bringing bent arms forward in fist position, etc. They move fast. Repeat L then R.

8   b.   Jog—do eight back to column formation facing front.

216   Repeat whole routine from beginning.

120   Repeat routine from beginning to, and including, Jumping Jack and Lunge.

Ending

Jump and full turn.

ROUTINE NUMBER 7: Aerobic Exercise (Polley 1978)

MUSIC: "Pine Apple Rag"

TIME: 2:35 Minutes

BASIC ACTION INCLUDES: Jogs, Sunshine Circle, Coordinator, Sunshine Jog, Half Breast Stroke, Skier, Back Kicks, Jump Kicks, Knee Push, Heel Hit, Flapper touch, Charleston Disco.

STARTING FORMATION: Alternate columns facing instructor.

INTRODUCTION: Begin jogs on the first note of the music. Do all skills on the right foot first unless instructed differently.

Counts

32   a.   Jog—do sixteen facing front, eight clockwise or moving R in own small circle, eight counterclockwise or moving L in own circle.

Step Number 1

16   a.   Jumping Jacks—do four by jumping to a feet

AEROBIC EXERCISE

Jumping Jacks

Coordinator

Sunshine Jacks

Sunshine Jog

Half Breast Stroke

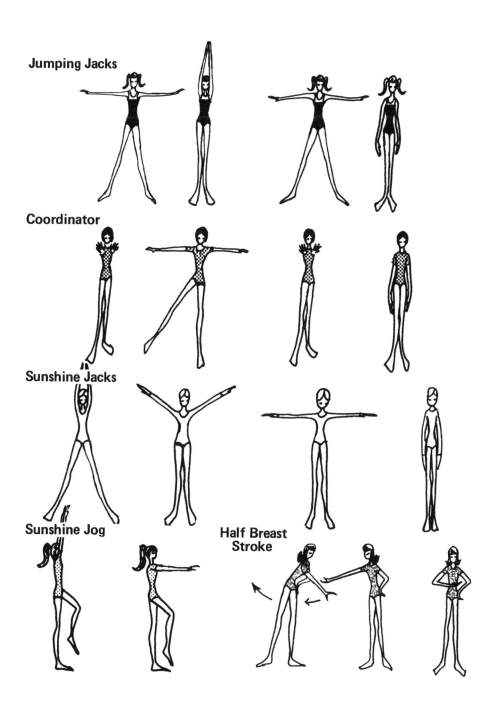

apart position (arms out to sides), jump bringing feet together (hands together overhead), jump feet apart (arms out to sides), jump feet together (arms down to sides).

16   b.   Coordinator—do four sets. Hop extending R foot forward (arms horizontal and forward), hop extending R foot out to the R side (arms horizontally out to the sides), hop extending R foot forward (arms horizontal and forward), jump bringing feet together (arms down to thighs). Repeat with the L, R then L.

Step Number 2

16   a.   Sunshine Jacks—do four (bringing arms overhead from center) as you jump feet apart, then jump three times with feet together (bringing arms out to the sides and down).

16   b.   Sunshine Jogs—do four sets. Jog R (extending arms above head in V position throwing head back), jog L (flexing arms with hands in fist position at shoulders). Jog R (extending arms horizontally forward). Jog L (flexing arms with hands in fist position at shoulders). Modification: Also extend to the side and down, two sets.

Step Number 3

8   a.   Half Breast Stroke—step to the side with L foot (sweep horizontally from L to R with R arm), body leaning forward at the waist. Repeat with the R arm.

8   b.   Jog—do eight beginning R in an individual small circle moving clockwise to the R.

16   c.   Repeat a and b with the L.

Step Number 4

16   a.   Skier—do twelve (R L R pause, L R L pause, etc.) by bringing R arm straight out to side and up overhead in fist position as L hand extends downward in fist position, as you jump sidewards to the R keeping the feet together.

16   b.   Back Kicks—do twelve (R L R pause, L R L pause, etc.) by jumping onto R extending L

Jog

Polka

Aerobic Taps

P.E. Slides

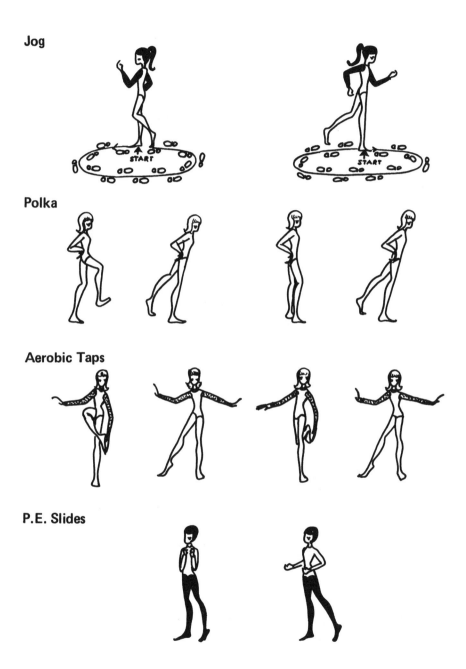

back (L arm up R down, fist position) jump onto L extending and R back (R arm up and L down, fist position).

Step Number 5

8	a.	Jump Kicks–do four; kicking legs straight forward (arms straight out to the sides).
8	b.	Vertical Jumps–do three clockwise in a small circle, clap facing front (wind up). Do three counterclockwise, clap facing front (unwind).
16	c.	Repeat a and b.
32		Repeat step number 4, Skier, Back Kicks.

Step Number 6, (form large circle)

16	a.	Jog–do sixteen in a large circle moving counterclockwise, beginning with R foot.
8	b.	Knee Push (facing center)–do two R, two L by hopping on L pushing R knee down with both hands, twice, etc.
8	c.	Heel Hit–hop as hit R heel (with R hand), touch R momentarily, hit R heel, step R. Repeat with L foot.

Step Number 7

16	a.	Jog–do sixteen clockwise beginning with R foot.
8	b.	Flapper Touch–do two (alternate R L) by extending R leg out to the side (bringing arms from a completely flexed position by shoulders with palms forward to an extended position horizontally to the front letting the hands flap forward). As you bring arms in by flexing them, close R foot to L. Repeat touch with the L.
8	c.	Heel Hit Turning–turn counterclockwise or L in own small circle by hitting R heel with R hand, touch R four times in between hits.
32		Repeat step number 6 a , b and c, Jog, Knee Push, Heel Hit.

Step Number 8

16	a.	Jog–do sixteen beginning with the R moving

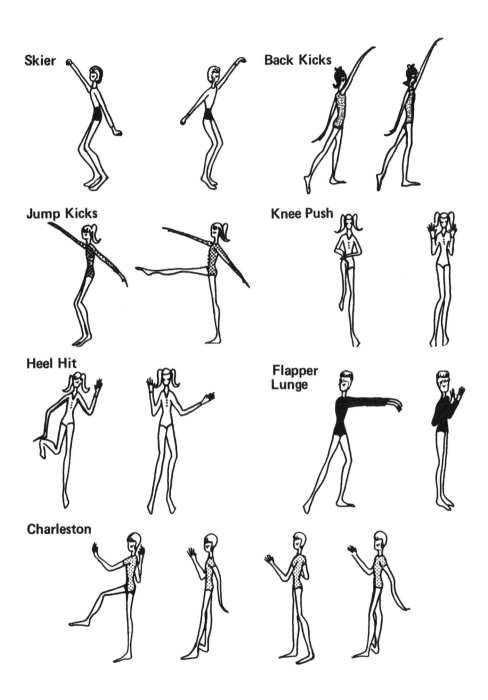

Skier

Back Kicks

Jump Kicks

Knee Push

Heel Hit

Flapper Lunge

Charleston

clockwise.

16   b.   Charleston Disco—do two basic disco steps by stepping forward L (facing center). Point R front, step back to place R, touch L back, arms extend forward in opposition, i.e., step forward L into place with R arm extending forward, flexed about ninety degrees, L arm back and flexed.

For style, when one foot is off the floor, the knees turn in; as the foot touches or steps, the feet turn outward. Action is like rubbing out a cigarette supposedly with both feet in opposition.

32   Repeat introduction. Jogs, moving into lines facing front.

32   Repeat step number 1. Jumping Jacks, Coordinator.

32   Repeat step number 2. Finish by bringing arms straight down to thighs instead of flexing the arms.

ROUTINE NUMBER 8: Aerobic Flight (Polley 1978)

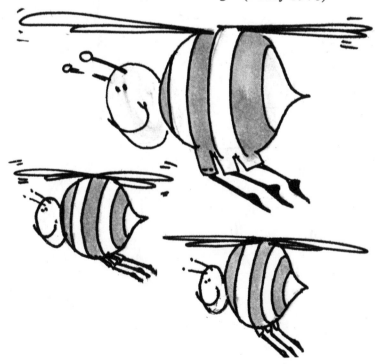

MUSIC: "Flight '76"

TIME: 3:29 Minutes

BASIC ACTION INCLUDES: Chasse, Kick Ball Change, Sugar Foot, Gallop, Cha Cha Chase, Cha Cha Cross Over, Suzi Q, Paddle Turns, Shorty George Boogie Move, Aerobic Jumps.

STARTING FORMATION: Large single circle facing center. Arms flexed ninety degrees at sides, hands in fist position.

INTRODUCTION: Eight measures, begin Chasse on first note of the music.

Counts

16   a.   Chasse—do eight slides moving counterclockwise, eight clockwise in a circle formation. On the first slide or Chasse, the arms pull backward in a ninety degree flexed position, moving forward on the second slide remaining flexed approximately ninety degrees, fist position, etc.

Break Number 1

16   a.   Kick Ball Change, Sugar Foot—do two Kick Ball Changes by kicking the R foot forward, step back R on ball of foot, step in place L while keeping some weight on R. Arms are behind the back, hands low. Do four Sugar Foots—step onto R one hundred eighty degrees to the R shifting weight, then step onto the L foot by twisting L one hundred eighty degrees, both feet turning in the same direction. Arms are down at the sides, flutter hands in a wave-like motion. Repeat all.

Step Number 1

16   a.   Gallop—move counterclockwise in the single large circle, Gallop four with R foot in front, then Gallop four with the L foot forward. Repeat four R, four L. Arms are diagonally extended. When R foot leads, R hand is low and L is high, etc.

16	b.	Pivot L one hundred eighty degrees on L and repeat four Gallop sets (R L R L) moving clockwise.

Break Number 2

16	a.	Paddle Turn begins facing center—do one R. In your own circle, execute turns like the Gallop except the weight is on the pivot foot (R when turning R) and the distance between the feet remains constant. Right arm is straight up, left is straight out to the side when turning to the R four steps with three touches. Skier L R L R. Repeat Paddle turn and Skier L.
16		Repeat break number 1, Kick Ball Change, Sugar Foot.
32		Repeat step number 1 a and b, Gallop.
16		Repeat break number 2, Paddle Turns.

Step Number 3 Practice facing front. Later, face in.

24	a.	Cha Cha Chase—to execute one set, step forward on L foot then pivot R one hundred eighty degrees, step L step R step L (quick cha cha cha) step forward R pivot L one hundred eighty degrees, step R step L step R (quick cha cha cha). Hands are on the hips in a turned under position. For style, look over shoulder, flick the foot. Repeat all twice.
8	b.	Full Turn—step forward L, shift to R as do a Full Turn R, step L step R step L in place (cha cha cha). Step back R step forward L, step R step L step R (cha cha cha). Hands are on hips but turned under. On the back step R, extend arms forward shoulder high, palms forward. On the cha cha cha the left hand is placed on the hip turned under, R arm is slightly flexed and extended forward, R index finger moves R L R, as head moves R L R, i.e., no, no, no!

Step Number 4 Practice facing front. Later, face in.

24	a.	Cha Cha Crossover—step L over R (L arm extended, index fingers extended downward, R

AEROBIC FLIGHT

Chasse'

Kick Ball Change

Sugar Foot

Gallop

Paddle Turn

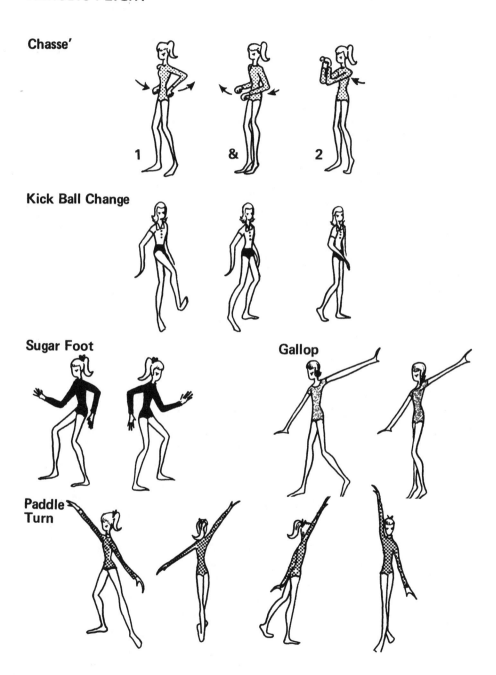

arm flexed ninety degrees). Step R in place, (R arm extended, L flexed) step L step R step L (extend L arm R arm flexed). Repeat to L side, step R over L, etc. Repeat the step L, R, L, R.

8   b.   Repeat step number 3 b, Full Turn.

Break number 3

16   Suzi Q—do eight R then eight L facing center of the large circle. Accomplish this by moving the feet together to the R one hundred eighty degrees, then moving the heels R one hundred eighty degrees, etc. Move the heels first when beginning Suzi Q's to the L. Arms are down near the sides, palms parallel to the floor, fingers out to sides, or do sixteen R.

32   Repeat step number 1 a and b, Gallop.

16   Repeat break number 2, Paddle Turns.

32   Repeat step number 3 a and b, Cha Cha Chase, Full Turn.

32   Repeat step number 4 a and b, Cha Cha Cross Over, Full Turn.

16   Repeat break number 3, Suzi Q.

32   Repeat step number 1 a and b, Gallop.

16   Repeat break number 2, Paddle Turns.

Ending

16   a.   Aerobic Jumps—do eight by jumping vertically, clap on the downbeat, arms flexed at a ninety degree angle pulling elbows backward, fist position obtained after the clap.

8   b.   Shorty George Boogie Move—do six with legs together by moving the knees to the R (R arm extended straight down, index fingers extended downward, L arm flexed ninety degrees) then move knees to L (L arm extended, R flexed). Do four moving body downward increasing the amount of flexion at the knees each move, then do two upward. Jump to a straddle stand, crossing arms as they open up to the high diagonal final position with feet apart.

Cha-Cha

Touch Full Turn

Push Step

Cha-Cha Crossover

Suzie-Q

Aerobic Jump

Shortie George Boogie

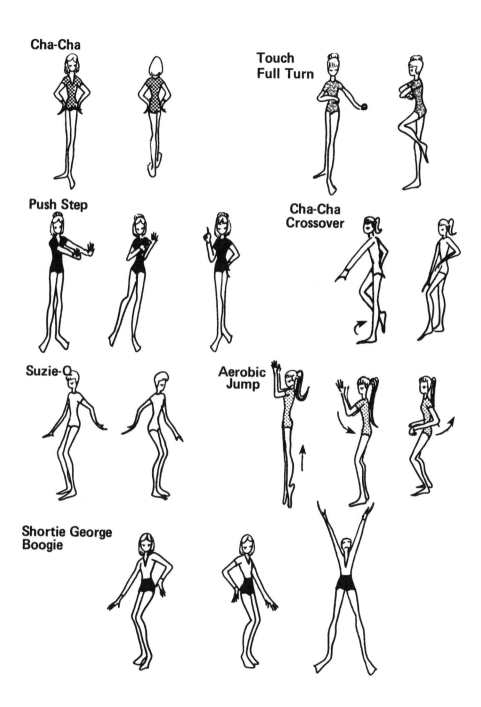

ROUTINE NUMBER 9: Snappy Jazz (Polley 1978)

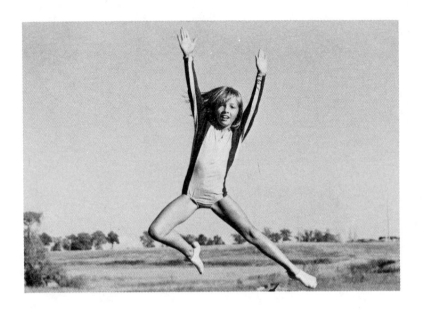

MUSIC: "Glad"

TIME: 1:45 Minutes

BASIC ACTION INCLUDES: Windshield Wiper, Jazz Two Steps, Sunshine Two Steps, Prance, Punch, Pivot Turns, Straight Kicks, Knee Hook, Scissor Kick, and Jazz Variety.

STARTING FORMATION: Alternate column formation. Stand with back to audience, feet apart, arms down at sides with fingers together.

INTRODUCTION: Wait seven counts. On count eight, bend L arm touching L hand behind head with fingers apart, L leg bends inward and R hand moves up to the hip.

Step Number 1

Counts

16   a.   Windshield Wiper—do eight (alternate R L etc.) bending legs inward. Extend L arm horizontally to the L with fingers spread, the palms facing away from audience while the head turns far L toward audience and R knee bends,

SNAPPY JAZZ

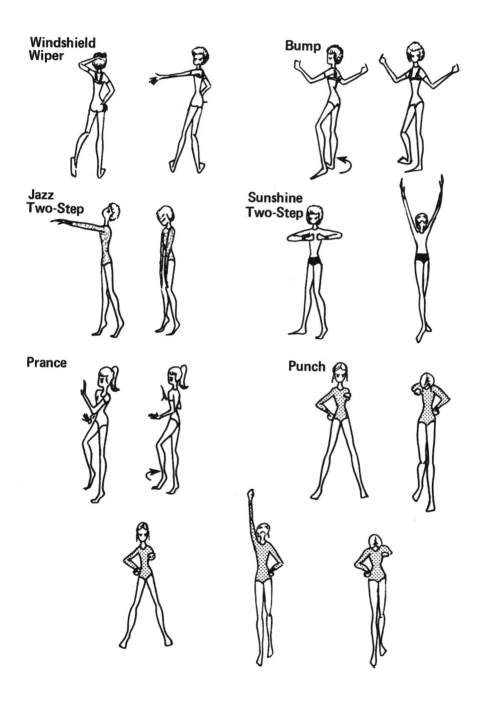

Windshield
Wiper

Bump

Jazz
Two-Step

Sunshine
Two-Step

Prance

Punch

R hand still on hip. As the R leg straightens, the L bends and the L hand touches the back of the head, eyes front.

16   b.   Bump—step ninety degrees with R foot to the L and toward the back (now your side is toward audience, feet still apart). Bump (individual) two R, two L, R, L, two R. Repeat beginning L, snap fingers only after second bump. L arm is forward as you bump to R while the R arm is back and out to the side, hands in snapping position.

Step Number 2, (move into own single, large circle moving counterclockwise).

16   a.   Two Steps—do eight (alternate R L etc.). To begin, step R close L step R, swinging the arms horizontally to the R on the step close, slap the thighs on the second step. Arms swing horizontally to the L on the second Two Step. Eye focus is high as the step begins. Drop head as hands slap thighs.

8   b.   Sunshine Two Steps—do two (R L). Step R to the R, close L, step R (thumbs in armpits) step back L (extend arms straight up, head back) step R in place (bring arms down, thumbs in armpits). Repeat to the L.

8   c.   Prance—do six (alternate R L R L R L), then do two Bumps R. The Prance is like marching, however, pivot on the supporting foot to give a twisting effect. Arms are flexed about one hundred thirty-five degrees with palms up toward audience and they move to the R as the R leg bends and to the L as the L leg bends. The L leg bends twice when beside R as hip bumps twice to the R. Index fingers extend downward, the L arm flexes as L leg bends.

Step Number 3

8   a.   Punch—step L to the side as you extend L arm horizontally in fist position and R arm comes to the hip in fist position (count one). Extend R arm forward in fist position bringing L to the

hip as you touch R foot behind L with leg extended (count two). Step R to the side as you extend L arm fist position, R hand to hip (count three). Extend R arm straight overhead, L hand comes to L hip as you touch L foot behind R with leg extended, head up (count four). Look down as you extend L arm horizontally forward in fist position, bringing R hand to hip (count five). Hold (counts six, seven, eight).

8   b.   Pivot Turns in a square—do four with the L foot. Step L forward and pivot ninety degrees to the R. Arms are extended downward, fingers together and upward—use a sweeping motion in front of the body from R to L as you pivot.

16   c.   Repeat a and b.

Step Number 4

16   a.   Kicks in a square moving counterclockwise—do four using R leg, i.e. Jump Kick R straight forward with arms extending straight overhead. Jump Hook R knee as you turn ninety degrees counterclockwise, arms extending straight down to the sides. Repeat Kicks in a square moving clockwise. Do four using L leg in like manner, the arm action being the same.

8   b.   Diagonally L: Jump Kick R in an extended position. Jump Knee Hook R, Jump Kick R leg in an extended position.
Front: Scissor Kick (jump onto R extending L, jump onto L extending R leg).

8   c.   Repeat step number 2 b, Prance.

Step Number 5

32   Repeat step number 3, Punch, Pivot Turns.

Step Number 6

32   Repeat step number 2, Two Steps, Prance.

Step Number 7

8   a.   Jazz Walk alternate rows—Odd rows: Step side L with L. Clap high diagonally L. Cross R foot over L. Clap low R back diagonally. Repeat.

**Pivot
Turns**

**Kick Knee,
Hook**

**Jazz
Walk**

**Jazz
Variety**

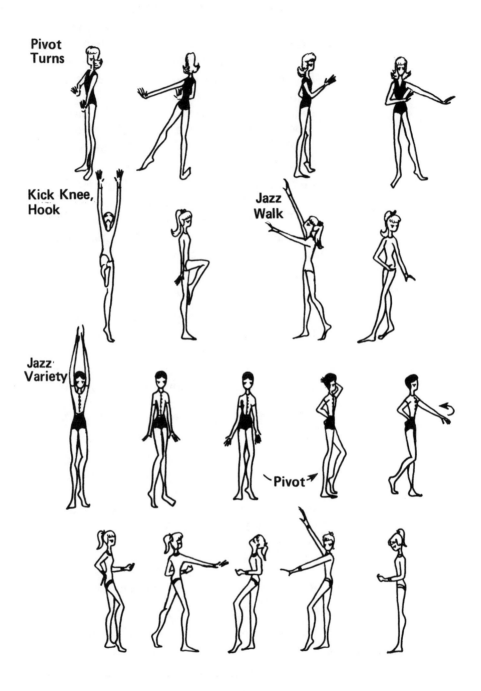

Pivot

Even rows: Shift weight to L foot at end of last step, then step side R with R. Clap high diagonally R. Cross L foot over R. Clap low back diagonally L. Repeat.

8   All Rows—pivot one hundred eighty degrees and repeat all facing away from audience.

4   b.   Jazz Variety—face audience, touch L beside R while bringing arms out to sides and up to clasp hands above head (sharply). Bring arms straight down with backs of hands toward audience. Bend R leg. Turn palms forward, bending L leg, pivot L (hold).

4   Moving ninety degrees to the L keeping L leg bent, R hand coming to R hip and L hand touching behind head (counts five, six). Bump L hip twice (counts seven, eight).

8   Step forward L as you make an outward horizontal curley Q with L hand, bringing arm flexed horizontally into waist in fist up position. Touch R foot beside L. Do a one hundred eighty degree horizontal sweep with R hand as you step forward R, then pivot one hundred eighty degrees, touch L foot beside R in a flexed position, bringing R arm in a horizontally flexed position to the waist in a fist up position. Lean body forward after turn, and straighten up body (sharp), head up on the pull in and touch (head up). Hold (counts five, six) til drum. On count seven, extend L arm horizontally front and R arm straight up (turn head L toward instructor or audience). Bring them down to waist—fist position (head down) as straighten L leg (count eight).

ROUTINE NUMBER 10: Beethoven's Special (Polley 1978)
MUSIC: "A Fifth of Beethoven"
TIME: 3:01 Minutes
BASIC ACTION INCLUDES: Triangle Touch, Criss Cross,

Paddle Turn, Suzi Q, Touch Step, Sugar Foot, Hustle Square, Train, Jazz Moves, Chasse.

STARTING FORMATION: Alternate columns facing instructor. Feet are together, head down, arms down at sides, hands on thighs.

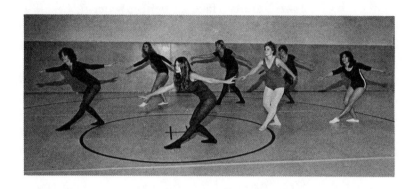

INTRODUCTION: Wait twenty-four counts with pauses and drum sound. Begin after third pick-up note.

Step Number 1

Counts

16   a.   Triangle Touch—touch R foot front, side, back, step forward with R. Touch L foot front, side, back, step forward with L. Repeat all. Arms remain down at sides, hands on thighs. R shoulder moves forward as you touch back R. L shoulder moves forward as L foot touches in back. On the fourth triangle, turn ninety degrees L as you step onto L foot.

16   b.   Triangle Touch Square—do four sets (alternate R L R L) in a square, moving counterclockwise. Do the step as above beginning with R foot. Turn ninety degrees on each step, the first triangle faces L, second one faces back, third one faces right, fourth faces front again. The last step L closes beside R.

Small Break

4   a.   Criss Cross—jump feet apart and flex arms, hands at shoulders in fist position. Pivot ninety

degrees R, drop hips and flex L leg, cross arms at chest and snap fingers. Next, rise up on toes facing front, pivot ninety degrees L, cross arms and snap.

4   Shift hips diagonally forward (hands cross), shift backward (forearms parallel), shift forward (hands cross). Close L back, arms are flexed, palms out at eye level.

16   b.   Suzi Q, Paddle Turn, Walk—do four Suzi Q's by turning toes R, moving heels R, turn toes R, move heels R. Hands are low with fingers up. Ball change four (ball R step L) times moving clockwise (if not facing in). Walk R L R touch L (clap). Walk L R L touch R (clap) to form large circle moving counterclockwise.

Step Number 2

      Chasse—do eight facing center, moving counterclockwise, eight clockwise in large circle. On the first slide or Chasse, the arms pull backward in a ninety-degree flexed position, moving forward on second slide flexed ninety degrees, fist position, etc. Snap, snap with R hand, flexing arm then extending it downward (pause in music), moving R knee inward twice.

   b.   Walk R L R touch L (snap), walk L R L touch R (snap) moving back to place to face front.

8   c.   Touch Touch Touch Step—touch R in back, touch R to side, touch R in back, step R. Repeat with L foot, etc. Shimmy the shoulders, or move arms R L and circle, etc.

Large Break   (interlude)

8   a.   Hustle Variety Square—walk back, three beginning R, then touch L and clap. Walk front, three beginning L, touch R and clap. Arms swing naturally at sides in opposition. Flex knees on the walks as in disco dancing.

   b.   Step side R, close L, step side R, touch L (moving R). Step side L, close R, step side L, touch R (moving L). Arms are flexed somewhat and move in opposition along the sides of the body.

BEETHOVEN'S SPECIAL

Triangle Touch

Criss-Cross   **Shift Hips**

Suzie-Q

Paddle Turn

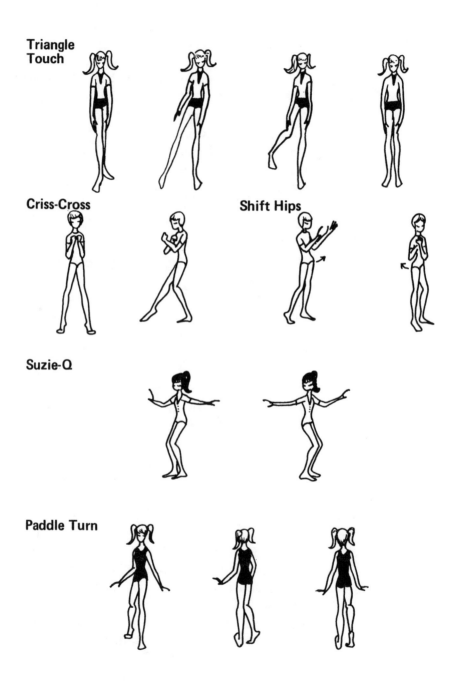

**Touch
Circle**

**Hustle-Square
Side-Steps**

**Funky
Chicken**

Train

Jazz Freak I

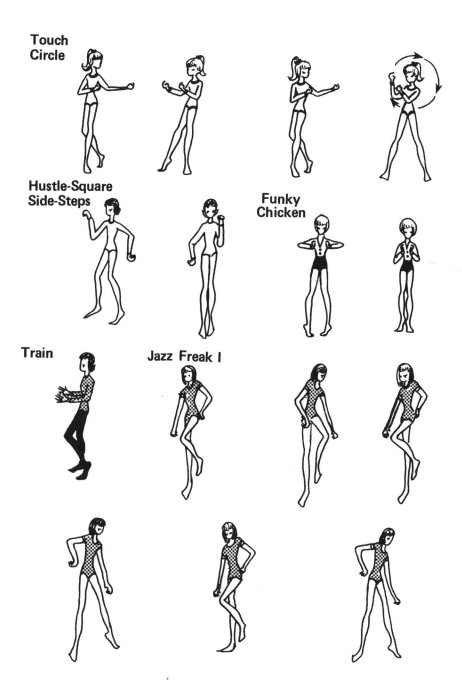

Fingers snap as you touch. R arm comes down, stepping R. L arm comes down stepping L.

4   c.   Jump back, hit heels together twice (thumbs in armpits, flap elbows twice). Pivot to L ninety degrees as kick R leg forward.

60   d.   Repeat a, b and c three times.

12   a.   Train—do three diagonal two steps to the side (alternate R L R) fist position. Arms circle forward twice on each two step (hands perpendicular to the ground).

2   b.   Jazz Freak I—bend L knee to R leg (R arm down, L arm flexed ninety degrees along side). Extend L leg out to side (L arm extends fist position toward L foot while R arm bend at a ninety degree angle, fist position).

2   c.   Bend L knee to R leg and move in this position from R to L to R, then extend to the L (arms extend downward alternating R L R L, the other being flexed).

16   d.   Repeat a, b and c. On pick-up notes, jump onto L extending R, ready for step number 1.

32   Repeat step number 1, Triangle Touch, Triangle Touch Square.

24   Repeat small break, Criss Cross, Suzi Q etc.

32   Repeat step number 2, Chasse, Walks, Touch Step.

Ending: Jazz Freak II

a.   Bring L leg to R knee (R arm down, L flexed ninety degrees along side), L leg moves L (L arm extends, R flexes), L leg moves R still at knee (R arm extends, L flexes), L leg extends to the side (L arm extends, R flexes), throw head back. Repeat all.

b.   Do three leg bend extensions (alternately extend arms R L R L R L). Step L next to R, step R to the side opening arms above head. Bring them around and slap thighs touching L foot in back, head down. Hold counts 6, 7, 8.

c.   Step forward L on the pick-up notes, R arm ex-

Jump Point

Jazz Freak II

Ending

tended by fourth pick-up note, shoulder high with palm forward, while L arm is completely flexed, palm forward at L shoulder. Pivot ninety degrees to R, R hand coming to R shoulder, the arm becoming completely flexed while L arm extends forward shoulder high with palm forward. Eye focus is directly ahead of hands. Extend R arm palm forward, while you flex L arm to L shoulder palm forward, bringing L leg flexed to R knee. Simultaneously turn head sharply to the L to face audience, left side of body remains toward the front.

FIVE BALLET POSITIONS

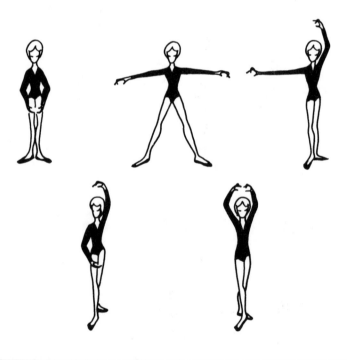

ROUTINE NUMBER 11: Music Box Dancer

MUSIC: "Music Box Dancer"

TIME: 3:17 Minutes

BASIC ACTION INCLUDES: Ballet Grapevine, Ballet Walks, Leg Swing, Pendulum Swings, Glissode Step Point, Fan Kicks.

INTRODUCTION: Wait for sixteen counts.

Step Number 1

Counts

16   a.   Ballet Grapevine—step R (arms out to the sides, second position). Cross L foot over R (bring L arm low across body) step R (L arm up, R out to side, third position). Point L to the L (turn hips L, arms in low second position). Repeat L, R, then L.

4   b.   Ballet Walk front—walk R L R point L forward. (Bring curved arms from low first to an overhead position or fifth, open hands somewhat as you point).

4   c.   Ballet Walk back—walk L R L point R forward. (Bring arms straight downward and back on the Walks).

8   d.   Repeat b and c.

Step Number 2

16   a.   Leg Swing—swing R leg forward (bring parallel straight arms to a forward horizontal position. Brush R foot back beside L then out to the R in one motion (arms come straight down then out to the sides). Step R beside L (bring arms down to sides). Repeat L, R, then L.

16   b.   Dance Circle—on the balls of your feet, step R close L step R, bring L foot through and forward (off the floor). As you drop R heel, bring R arm forward palm up, extending toward L foot. Repeat L, R, then L.

Step Number 3

32   a.   Pendulum Swings—with feet apart, shift weight as you swing parallel arms to the horizontal R

then swing L, full circle counterclockwise (do a step R close L step R). Swing parallel arms to the L etc. Repeat beginning L, R then L.

Small Break   (interlude)

16   On the feet; step R forward, step L forward beside L, step back R, step back L beside R. Arms are curved, fingers touching sides.

96   Repeat routine from the beginning.

16   Repeat small break (interlude).

96   Repeat routine again then add this new part.

Step Number 4

4   a.   Glissode Arabesque Saute—moving diagonally forward R—step R (arms out and low), close L (curve arms low first), step R hop R (R arm high diagonally R with L arm low diagonally back).

4   b.   Glissode Step Point—moving diagonally backward L—step L (arms out to sides), close R (curved arms low first), step L (L arm out, R curved in low first), point R (L arm high diagonal L, R flexed in front of chest, body leaning forward).

24   Repeat step number 4 three more times.

Step Number 5

32   Fan Kick Step—step R (arms out) kick L leg across body L to R from low to high (arms move from low first to open overhead). Glissade or step L close R, step L, cross R over L full turn (arms low and curved, fingers touching thighs). Step L Fan Kick R etc. Repeat Fan Kick L then R.

16   Repeat step number 1, Ballet Grapevine only til the end.

MUSIC BOX DANCER

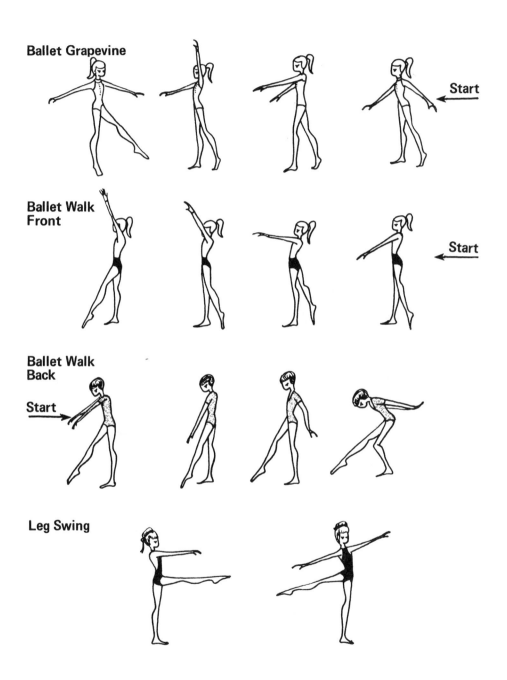

Ballet Grapevine

Start

Ballet Walk Front

Start

Ballet Walk Back

Start

Leg Swing

Dance Circle

Pendulum Swings

Interlude

Glissode

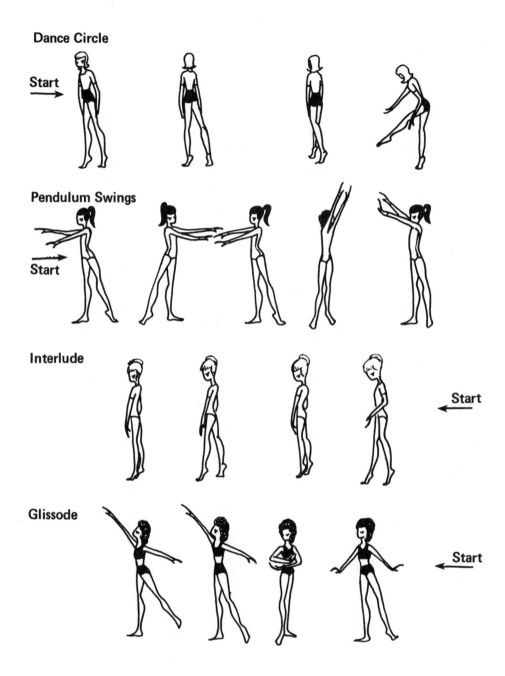

Start

Start

Start

Start

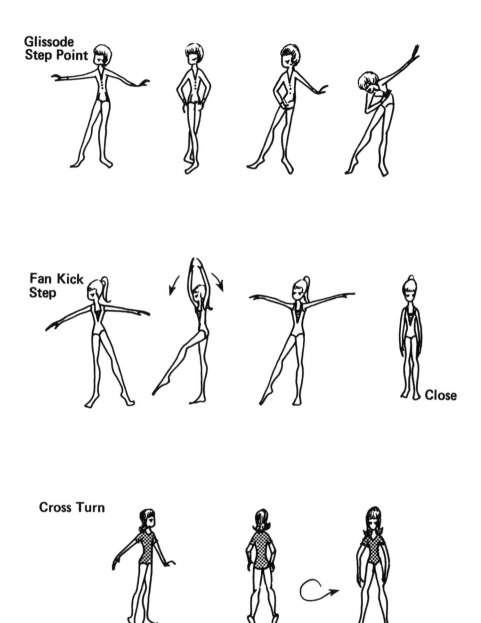

Glissode Step Point

Fan Kick Step

Close

Cross Turn

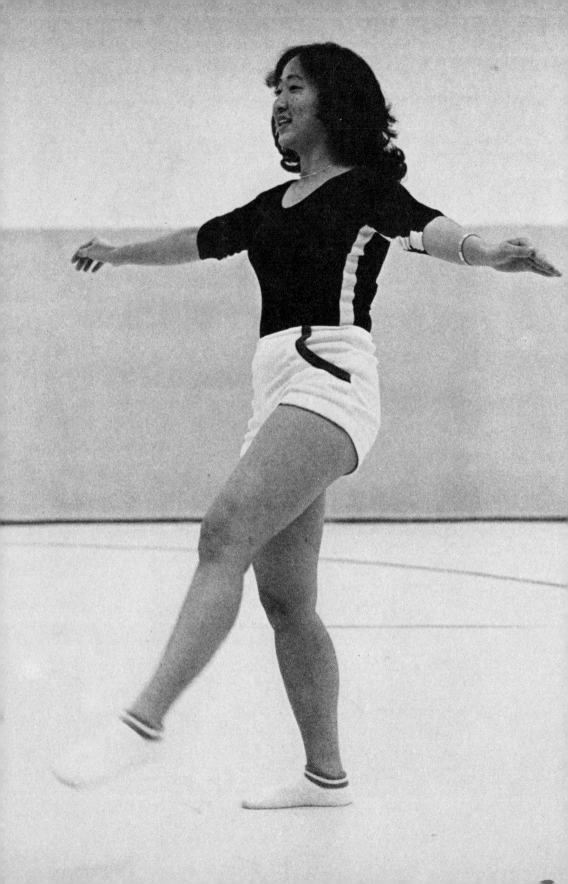

ROUTINE NUMBER 12: Disco Stomp

MUSIC: "We are Family" or almost any disco song

TIME: 2:18 Minutes, "Shame" is provided.

BASIC ACTION INCLUDES: Side Strut, Three Step Turn, Suzi Q, Touch-Step-Stomp, Windmill.

STARTING FORMATION: Three or four columns facing the instructor, alternating female, male, female, male, etc. The directions are written for the males. Females should go the opposite direction using the opposite foot throughout the routine.

Step Number 1

Counts

24 a. Side Strut—step R to the R, close L, step R, touch L beside R (clap). Step L to the L, close R, step L, touch R (clap). Repeat twice.

8 b. Three Step Turn—step R to the R, step clockwise one hundred eighty degrees onto L, step around R to face the front. Touch L beside R (clap). Repeat L.

Step Number 2

16 a. Suzi Q—move toes R, heels R, toes R, heels R. Repeat L, R then L.

6 b. Touch-Step-Stomp—do two sets. Touch R to the side (R shoulder forward). Close R, touch L to the side (L shoulder forward). Close, stomp, stomp with R foot.

6 Repeat b. On second stomp extend R arm diagonally R. Girls may look back at the guy behind them on L touches.

4 c. Windmill—bring arm down to the horizontal, down lower, down to low diagonal, clap.

Repeat steps for as long as you like. This routine is great for large groups. If you find it easier for both males and females do the Touch-Step-Stomp step on the R (males' part), do so. You may also do the Windmill on the R (males' part) for the whole group.

DISCO STOMP

Side Strut

3-Step Turn   **Suzie-Q**

**Stomp
Step**

Ending

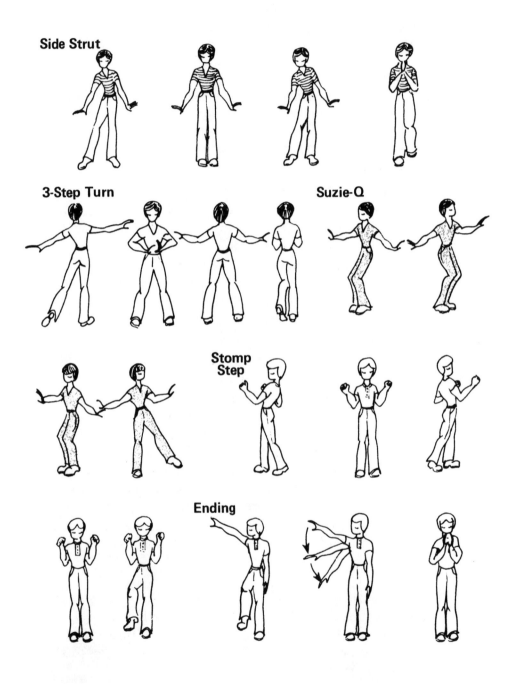

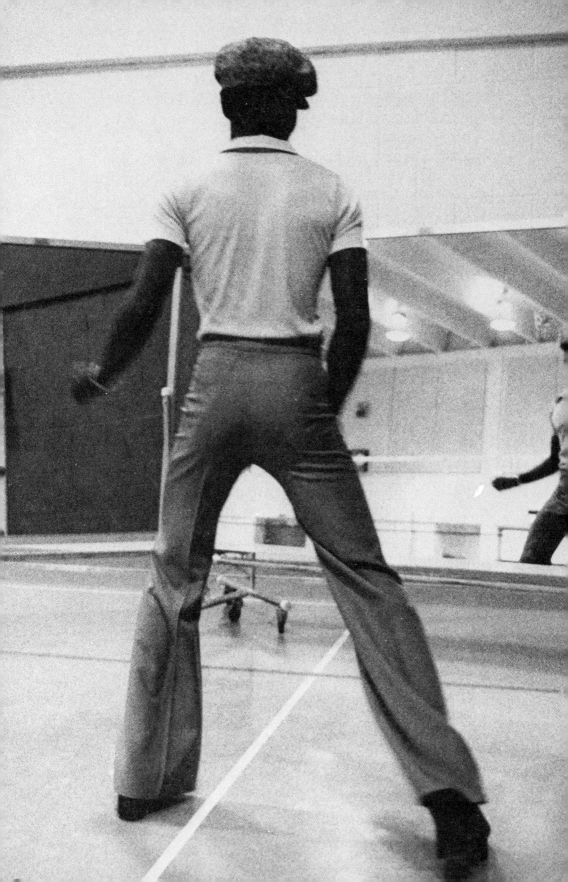

ROUTINE NUMBER 13: Cooldown with Nadia (Polley 1978)

MUSIC: "Nadia's Theme"

TIME: 2:50 Minutes

BASIC ACTION INCLUDES: Toe Rise, Sunshine Circles, Two Step Kick, Ballet Square, Rainbow Turn, Horizontal Pulls, Step Cross, Ballet Touch.

STARTING FORMATION: Alternate columns facing the instructor.

INTRODUCTION: Wait eight counts.

Step Number 1

Counts

16   a.   Toe Rise-Arm Lift—rise slowly up on the toes, then down, while simultaneously sweeping the R arm from next to the body, out to the side and overhead. Continue moving the arm by starting downward and out to finish down at the R side. Repeat with the L arm in like manner, then R and L, etc. Eyes should focus on the moving hand.

16   b.   Rainbows (body)—as you step to the side with L foot, begin to circle the R arm (extended) across. the front of the body from low to high (L to R) making a complete circle clockwise coming to rest on R thigh. R heel lifts when R arm is on L side of body. Next, with the L arm from down at the side, circle the L arm across body from low to high (R to L) making a complete circle counterclockwise coming to rest on the L thigh. L heel lifts when L arm is on R side of body. Repeat all. Close L foot to R on last L arm circle as the L hand comes to rest on L thigh.

Step Number 2

32   a.   Sunshine Circle—bring arms from first ballet position (arms curved low with fingers touching in front of body) up to fifth position (overhead). Separating the arms, they pass through second position (out to the sides). Bend the trunk forward with arms out to the sides then

sweep fingers downward over toes. Straighten trunk slowly, keeping arms curved and fingers touching, ready to begin the arm circle again. Eyes follow arm movement.

Step Number 3

16 a. Two Step Kick—step forward R, close L step R kick L. Repeat L, then R, L. The arms extend easily to the R when executing the Two Step on the R. On the kick L, the L arm extends out to the L side, R arm staying R.

16 b. Step Step Step Touch—first step back R, step back L, step back R, extend and touch L foot out to the side. After the steps, do a small circle (scoop) with the hands toward yourself, then extend palms toward L foot in a pushing motion as that foot is extended. On the last touch R, step on it turning body ninety degrees R.

Step Number 4

16 a. Rainbow Turn—begin with a step forward on the L (L side to audience), pivot one hundred eighty degrees to the R with weight on both feet, (extend R arm forward and up, making a full circle), (the L arm starting when R is straight up). Close L foot to R. Repeat stepping forward L pivoting one hundred eighty degrees R, close L foot to R. Step forward L as you turn the body ninety degrees to face audience, pivot R one hundred eighty degrees R, close L. Step forward L facing back (back to audience) pivot R one hundred eighty degrees R, close L foot to R, end facing audience again, having completed four fancy "to the rear" turns. Arms are the same for each Rainbow Turn.

16 b. Ballet Square—step front R close L, step side R close L, step back R touch L, step L close R. Step front L close R, step side L close R, step back L touch R, step R close L. Use the same arm as lead leg and in that direction, extending the arm waist high. Exception: Swing arm for-

COOL DOWN WITH NADIA

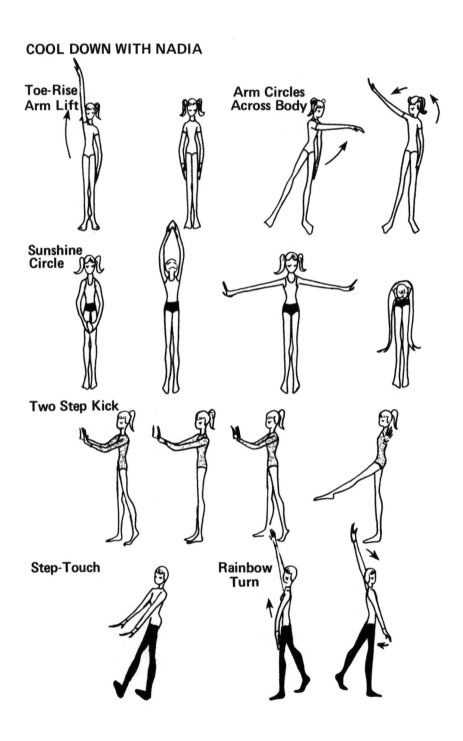

Toe-Rise
Arm Lift

Arm Circles
Across Body

Sunshine
Circle

Two Step Kick

Step-Touch

Rainbow
Turn

Ballet Square

Horizontal Pulls

Step-Cross

Ballet Touch

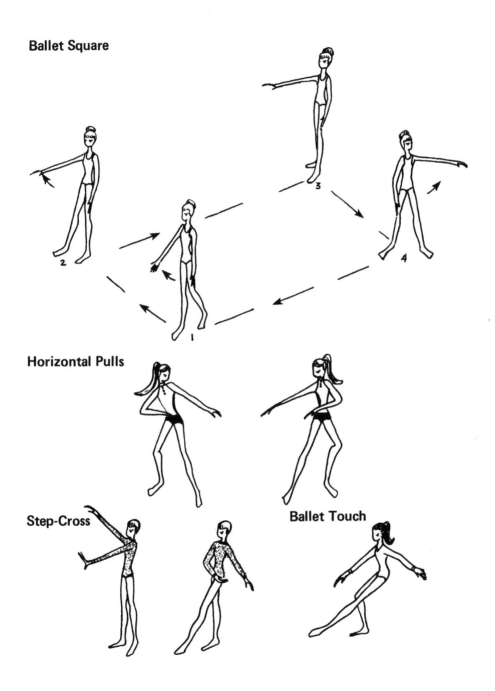

ward as step backward. Eyes follow arm movement.

Step Number 5

16   a.   Horizontal Pulls—pull the arms horizontally with arms flexed to the R (R leg flexed as steps out to the side on the first arm pull). The L leg is flexed as the weight shifts toward the L, arms pulling horizontally to the L, etc. Do five more horizontal pulls beginning L.

16   b.   Step Cross—moving R, step on the R (arms diagonally high R), cross L over R (arms low L). Repeat twice. Step R turning ninety degrees R, close L (now facing back, back toward the audience). Do three Step Crosses moving R, turn to end facing front or toward the audience. Eye focus is on the hands.

32   Repeat step number 1 a and b. Toe Rise, Arm Circles Across Body.

Ending

8   a.   Ballet Touch—do an arm circle with both arms as in step number 2. After bringing arms out to the sides, execute a Ballet Touch, i.e., point L foot forward on the floor, extend R arm forward nearly touching L foot while flexing R leg and moving L arm back low and straight. Eye focus is on L foot, keep chest up. Hold four counts, then stand by bringing L foot to R, arms to sides.

ROUTINE NUMBER 14: Cooldown with Dr. Z

MUSIC: "Lara's Theme from Dr. Zhivago"

TIME: 2:53 Minutes

BASIC ACTION INCLUDES: Walks, Step Point, Two Step, Body Bends, Leg Swings, Lunge.

STARTING FORMATION: Alternate columns facing teacher.

INTRODUCTION: Wait for the short run, then begin on the first note of the theme.

Step Number 1
Counts

8   a.   Walk—do three (R L R) moving forward then point L back. Arms move parallel and forward, from down at the sides on the first step to diagonally overhead on the point.
Walk—do three (L R L) moving backward then point R front. Arms move straight downward on the walk, extending backward on the point.

8   b.   Repeat a, Walk etc.

8   c.   Moving sideward, step R (arms out and low). Close L (arms curved low) step diagonally R and point L diagonally back as you extend R arm diagonally forward. The L hand is low and extended backward (low arabesque). Repeat to the L.

8   d.   Step R (arms low and out) cross L over R (arms curved low in first position). Pivot, turning completely around as you extend arms curved overhead (fifth position) then open to sides and down. Step L, cross R over L and turn completely around to the L using the arms in like manner.

Step Number 2

4   Two Step—do one R bringing L arm up from side to curved position overhead, Two Step L with R arm in a curved position overhead. to sides and down.

4   Two Step—R bringing L arm up from side to curved position overhead, Two Step L with R arm in a curved position overhead.

8   Leg Swings—swing R forward, brush close then swing immediately to the side, close R. Swing L forward, brush close then immediately swing leg out to the side, close L. Arms swing parallel and forward with leg, then out to the sides as leg swings out. Repeat leg swing (forward, brush close then out to side, lunge R (L arm full circle counterclockwise), close R.

COOLDOWN WITH DOCTOR Z

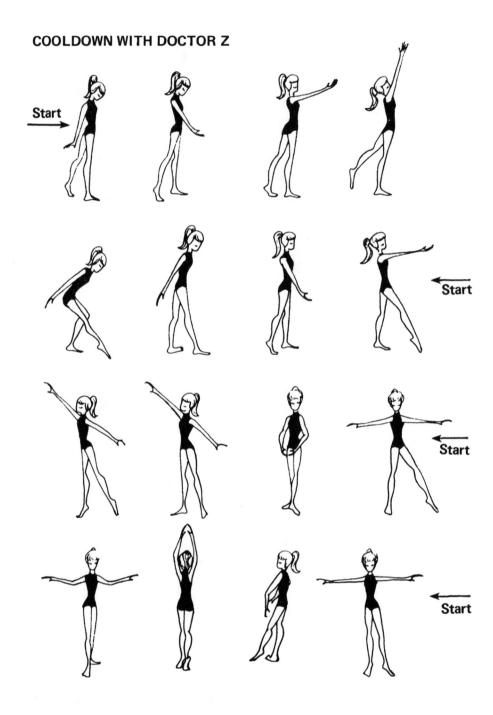

Start

Start

Start

Start

Start

Two Steps

Start

Start

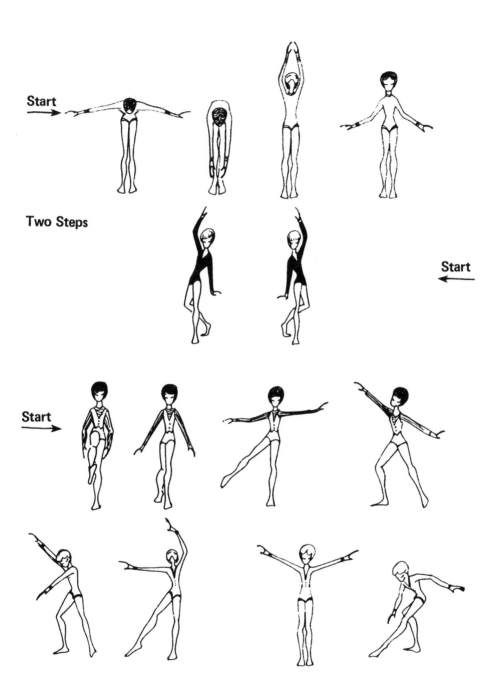

16   b.   Repeat a, Body Bend.
            Repeat step number 1 a, b, c and d, Walk etc.
            Repeat step number 2 a and b, Body Bend, etc.
            Repeat step number 1, Walks etc.

Ending

            Extend L foot forward pointing the toes, flex-
            ing the R leg while bringing the arms straight
            backward. Eye focus is on L foot.

ROUTINE NUMBER 15: Summer Cooldown

MUSIC: "Theme from A Summer Place"

TIME: 2:26 Minutes

BASIC ACTION INCLUDES: Walks, Slow Kicks, Three Step
        Turn, Coordinator, Horizontal Pulls, Glissode Ara-
        besque, Glissode Attitude, Glissode Cross Turn,
        Body Bends, Ballet Touch.

STARTING FORMATION: Alternate columns facing in-
        structor.

INTRODUCTION: Wait for eight counts.

Step Number 1

Counts

    32   a.   Walks—do three moving forward (R L R),
            kick L forward (bring curved arms above head,
            open out to the sides and down—first, fifth,
            second and resting position). Do three moving
            backward (L R L), point R forward (arms ex-
            tend low in back). Repeat Walks (three times
            total), turning ninety degrees R after the for-
            ward point, forming a square.
            Variation: Use a step close step kick for the
            walks.

Small Break

    8   a.   Glissode Arabesque—do one moving R then
            one moving L (step R close in front L, step R
            diagonal scale) or step R close L step R, point.

Large Break

    8   a.   Three Step Turn—(R L R) moving R, touch L.

Three Step Turn—(L R L) moving L, touch R.

1-2   b.   Coordinator—step on the R turning ninety degrees R, extending L leg back, the L arm extending horizontally forward, while the R arm is out to the R side.

3-4   Shift weight to the back foot (L), switch arms (R forward L back).

5-6-7   Circle arms downward toward each other, continuing on around, each moving away and in own circle, ending in starting position with L arm forward, and weight on the R foot.

8   Turn ninety degrees L to face front, arms to the sides, feet together.

Step Number 2

24   Repeat step number 1 doing the Walks facing front, side, and back only.

4   Step R to R, close L facing to the side, step R to R, close L facing front thus finishing the clockwise square.

Step Number 3

16   a.   Horizontal Pulls—do five (slow R, slow L, fast R L R pause) by pulling the arms horizontally with arms flexed to the R (R leg flexed as it steps out to the side on first arm pull). The L leg is flexed as the weight shifts toward the L, arms pulling horizontally to the L, etc. Repeat five Horizontal Pulls beginning L.

8   b.   Glissode Attitude—do one moving R, then one moving L. Step R, close L in front, step R lift L leg, waist high, in flexed position with knee out. The arms are in third with R overhead and L out horizontally to the side.

8   c.   Glissode Cross Turn—do one moving R then one moving L by stepping R, close L in front, step R, cross L over turning R one full turn, (arms curved overhead, out to the side, then down).

16   d.   Body Bends—with arms out to the sides, bend forward and sweep the hands in front of the

SUMMER COOLDOWN

Walks

Start

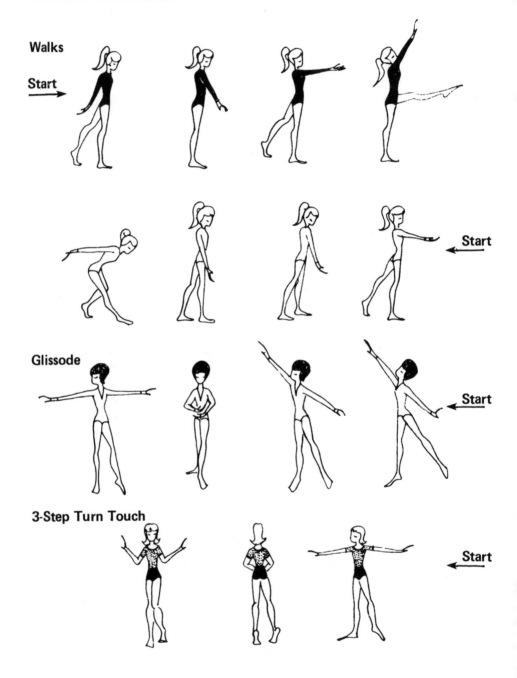

Glissode

3-Step Turn Touch

Coordinator

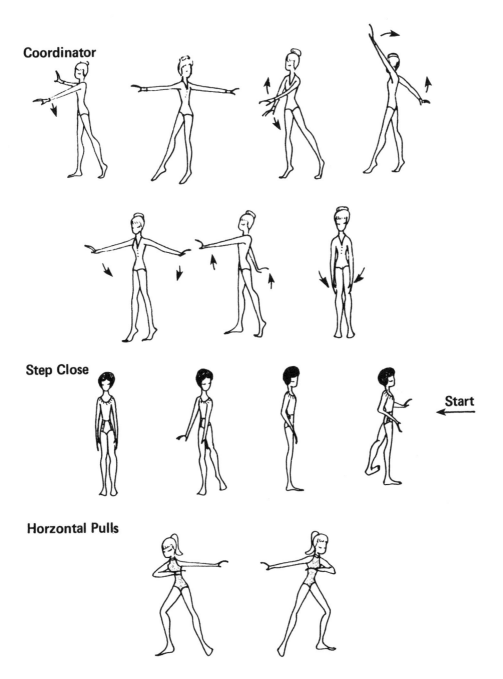

Step Close

Start

Horzontal Pulls

feet. Straighten up, bringing the curved arms
forward and overhead, opening out to the sides.
Repeat. Bring the L foot forward, flexing the R
(extending the R arm toward the L foot while
the L arm extends low in back) to Pose.

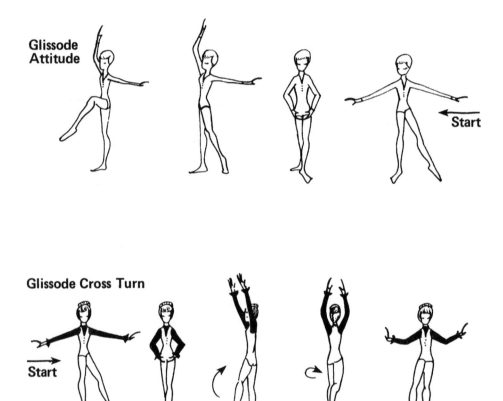

**Glissode
Attitude**

Start

Glissode Cross Turn

Start

Circle Arms

Pose

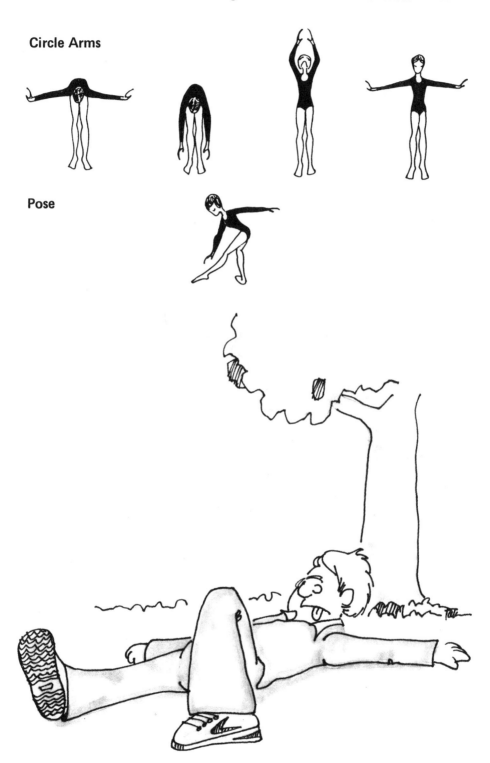

Part Four
Helpful Extras

TWELVE-WEEK BLOCK PLAN

This is just a guide. You are the experts. Modify this Program in light of your needs. Your comments will be appreciated. The speed of progression is dependent upon age, experience, size of group and leadership. If you are a rookie, this should prove helpful. Remember to employ the Principle of Continuous Movement and strive for no more than one minute between routines. If you don't have an Aerobics Unit per se, teach a routine to serve as the warm-up for other activities. Soon you'll have the confidence and student support to have Aerobic Dance put into the curriculum.

*FIRST WEEK

Session One
Record Resting Heart Rate
Introduction-Dance Aerobics
Warm-up by Stretching 5 min.
Teach the Pa. Hustle
Take the Cardiovascular Test
Teach Steps 1 & 2 Dance Variety
Teach Steps 1-3 Nadia's Cooldown.
Check Recovery Rate.
Encourage this habit

Session Two
Explain & figure Target Zones
Review Session One
Teach Chocolate Hustle
Teach Steps 3 & 4 Dance Variety
Teach Step 4 Nadia's Cooldown

Session Three (Your choice)
Review Session Two or
Have a lecture/discussion session
Try brisk walking or cycling

*SECOND WEEK

Session One
Discuss Aerobics
Warm-up Stretching
Do Pa. Hustle
Chocolate Hustle
Teach Bus Stop
Finish Dance Variety
Finish Nadia's Cooldown

Session Two
Repeat last Session
Teach Steps 1-3 Navy Special
Do Nadia's Cooldown

Session Three
Review Session Two
Lecture/discussion
or Swim with a friend

Check to see if you are in the Target Zone by taking Working Heart Rate after every one or two Aerobic Dances each session. *General* Target Zone limits are: 220 - age = _____,
X .70 & X .85.

*THIRD WEEK

Session One
Warm-up Stretching
Do Pa. Hustle
Chocolate Hustle
Bus Stop
Practice then teach
Steps 4 & 5 Navy Special
Practice then teach Steps 1 & 2
of Beethoven's Special
Do Nadia's Cooldown

Session Two
Repeat last Session
Finish teaching Navy Special
Teach Break & Step 3 Beethoven's
Do Nadia's Cooldown

Session Three
Review Session Two
Have lecture /discussion Session
or go cycling

*FOURTH WEEK

Session One
Warm-up Stretching
Do Pa. Hustle
Chocolate Hustle
Bus Stop
Do Dance Variety
Navy Special
Finish teaching Beethoven's
Do Nadia's Cooldown

Session Two
Repeat Session One
Teach Roller Coaster
Do Nadia's Cooldown

Session Three
Review Session Two
Play racquetball

*FIFTH WEEK

Session One
Warm-up Stretching
Do Disco Lines
Review Roller Coaster
Do Dance Variety
Navy Special
Teach Steps 1 & 2 of
Aerobic Jog
Do Beethoven's Special
Nadia's Cooldown

Session Two
Repeat Session One
Teach Steps 3 & 4 of
Aerobic Jog
Teach Steps 1 & 2 Dr. Z
Do Nadia's Cooldown

Session Three
Review Session Two
Have lecture/discussion
Play tennis or racquetball

*SIXTH WEEK

Session One
Take Dr. Cooper's 1.5 mile
Run Test
Cooldown with Dr. Z
Do Nadia's Cooldown

Session Two
Warm-up Stretching
Do the Disco Lines
Do Dance Variety
Navy Special
Review Steps 3 & 4
of Aerobic Jog
Do Beethoven's
Practice then finish Dr. Z
Do Nadia's Cooldown

Session Three
Review Session Two
Go jogging with a friend

*SEVENTH WEEK

Session One
Warm-up Stretching
Do Chocolate Hustle
Teach Hot Disco Combo
Do Dance Variety
Navy Special
Aerobic Jog
Beethoven's
Teach Steps 1-3 Music
Box Dancer
Do Dr. Z.s Cooldown

Session Two
Repeat Session One
Finish Music Box Dancer
Do Dr. Z's Cooldown

Session Three
Review Session Two
Lecture/discussion
Go cross-country skiing

*EIGHTH WEEK

Session One
Warm-up Stretching
Do Chocolate Hustle
Hot Disco Combo
Dance Variety
Navy Special
Aerobic Jog
Beethoven's
Music Box Dancer
Cooldown with Dr. Z

Session Two
Repeat Session One
Teach Steps 1 & 2 of
Summer Cooldown

Session Three
Review Session Two
Go jogging with a friend

*NINTH WEEK

Session One
Warm-up Stretching
Do Hot Chocolate
Hot Disco Combo
Repeat Dance Variety
Aerobic Jog
Teach Steps 1 & 2 of
Aerobic Exercise
Do Beethoven's Special
Music Box Dancer
Practice Summer Cooldown

Session Two
Repeat Session One
Teach Steps 3-5 Aerobic
Exercise
Finish teaching Summer
Cooldown

Session Three
Repeat Session Two
Have lecture/discussion
or go cross-country skiing

*TENTH WEEK

Session One
Warm-up Stretching
Do Chocolate Hustle
Hot Disco Combo
Dance Variety
Aerobic Jog

Finish teaching Aerobic
Exercise
Do Beethoven's Special
Music Box Dancer
Summer Cooldown

Session Two
Repeat Session One
Teach Steps 1 & 2 of
Aerobic Flight
Do Summer Cooldown

Session Three
Repeat Session Two
Do rope skipping

*ELEVENTH WEEK

Session One
Warm-up Stretching
Do Hot Disco Combo
Dance Variety
Aerobic Jog
Finish Teaching Aerobic
Flight
Do Beethoven's Special
Teach Steps 1 & 2 of
Snappy Jazz
Do Music Box Dancer
Summer Cooldown

Session Two
Repeat Session One
Teach Steps 3 & 4 of
Snappy Jazz
Do Summer Cooldown

Session Three
Repeat Session Two
Have lecture/discussion
Go jogging with a friend

*TWELFTH WEEK

Session One
Warm-up Stretching
Do Beethoven's Special
Finish Snappy Jazz
Take Efficiency Test, compare
Do Music Box Dancer
Summer Cooldown

Session Two
Check Resting Heart Rate
Review for Quiz
Take Dr. Cooper's 1.5 mile
Test. Compare

Session Three
Tie up loose ends
Mention next Session dates
Take written test
Check written test

CARDIOVASCULAR EFFICIENCY TEST
FOR GIRLS AND WOMEN

Standard step tests provide an index of cardiovascular efficiency, advantageously used during inclement weather or where running tracks are unavailable.

Skubic and Hodgkins obtained data from more than two thousand junior and senior high school girls from fifty-five secondary schools, and from two thousand three hundred sixty women from sixty-six colleges. The test successfully differentiated among the sedentary, active, and well-trained subjects (reliability coefficient .82 using test/re-test method). Mixed groups should use the Harvard Step Test from same source.

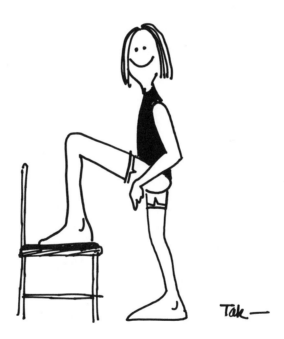

Testing Procedure: 1) Subjects face the step up bench or bleacher eighteen to twenty inches high. Command: Say, "Ready, go. Up, two, three, four, up two, three, four" etc. 2) Maintain the exercise for three minutes. 3) Take the pulse rate at the carotid artery, counting from one to one and one-half minutes after exercise. 4) If a subject becomes exhausted, she should sit down.

Scoring: The following formula is employed in computing subject's cardiovascular efficiency score:

$$\text{Efficiency Score} = \frac{\text{Number of seconds completed X 100}}{\text{Recovery pulse X 5.6}}$$

Example: A junior high school girl exercises for the full three minutes (one hundred eighty seconds). Her recovery pulse count measured from one to one and one-half minutes after exercise is fifty-five. Her cardiovascular efficiency score is:

$$\text{Efficiency Score} = \frac{180 \text{ X } 100}{5.6 \text{ X } 55} = \frac{18{,}000}{308} = 58.4 \text{ or } 58$$

NORMS: CARDIOVASCULAR EFFICIENCY TEST

	Junior H.S.	Senior H.S.	College
Excellent	72 - 100	71 - 100	71 - 100
Very Good	62 - 71	60 - 70	60 - 70
Good	51 - 61	49 - 59	49 - 59
Fair	41 - 50	40 - 48	39 - 48
Poor	31 - 40	31 - 39	28 - 38
Very Poor	0 - 30	0 - 30	0 - 27

Source: *Practical Measurements for Evaluation in Physical Education.* Copyright © 1974 by Barry Johnson and Jack Nelson, Burgess Publishing Company, Minneapolis. Reprinted by permission.

DESIRABLE WEIGHT RANGES

Height	Weight (Women)	Weight (Men)
5' 0"	85 - 100	
5' 1"	90 - 105	
5' 2"	95 - 110	105 - 123
5' 3"	100 - 115	110 - 128
5' 4"	105 - 120	115 - 134
5' 5"	110 - 125	120 - 139
5' 6"	115 - 130	125 - 145
5' 7"	120 - 135	130 - 150
5' 8"	125 - 140	135 - 156
5' 9"	130 - 145	140 - 161
5'10"	135 - 150	145 - 167
5'11"	140 - 155	150 - 172
6' 0"	145 - 160	155 - 178
6' 1"		160 - 183
6' 2"		165 - 190

This is the table I use, representing desirable weights. Remember that you can fit into the correct category and still lack muscle tone and cardiovascular fitness. The scientific community prefers body fat measurements.

Rather than having an almost fanatical desire to weigh exactly what the charts dictate, view them merely as a guide. They can be misleading. There is much more to fitness than weight. As you know, adipose tissue is only one-third as heavy as muscle, so a person can be obese (according to percent of body fat) and still not appear fat according to the charts.

Concerning weight, both men and women tend to lie to themselves, but in different ways. According to Charles T. Kuntzleman, national director for the Y.M.C.A. Fitness-Finders program, many women who are small-framed claim the medium frame as they gain weight. This provides them with an additional nine to eleven pounds. Whereas, when men have been gaining weight, they stick to the same frames, but convince themselves that they have been growing taller over the years, which allows them four or five extra pounds.

At least half of the body fat is stored directly beneath the skin, so by measuring the fold produced when the skin and the tissue are firmly grasped, it is possible to get an idea of the amount present. The triceps (back of the upper arm) and suprailiac (hip) fat measurements are taken on women. In addition to these, men are measured according to the sub-scapular (upper back) and the biceps (front of the arm). Relating these measurements to percent of body fat, then to actual weight, a person can determine how many pounds, if any, he or she needs to lose.

However, the common person doesn't make use of the caliper procedure, although it is more valid than the charts. Reasons include the lack of information and the cost of calipers (over one hundred dollars). Breakthroughs are coming, though. Plastic calipers priced from five dollars ninety-five cents to twenty dollars are now available.

In general, nineteen percent body fat is standard for men, twenty-two or twenty-three for women. Cosmetically, fifteen percent is used for men, eighteen or nineteen percent being desirable for women. You may wonder about runners. Although they come in every description, good runners are never fat. Male runners usually have less than ten percent body fat, women below twenty percent.

SAFETY PRECAUTIONS:
WARNINGS AND WHAT TO DO ABOUT THEM

Symptom: Abnormal heart action; e.g.—pulse becoming irregular—fluttering, jumping or palpitations in chest or throat—sudden burst of rapid heartbeats—sudden very slow pulse when a moment before it had been on target (immediate or delayed).

Cause: Extrasystoles (extra heart beats), dropped heart beats, or disorders of cardiac rhythm. This may or may not be dangerous and should be checked out by a physician.

Remedy: Consult physician before resuming exercise program. He may provide medication to temporarily eliminate the problem and allow you to safely resume your exercise program, or you may have a completely harmless kind of cardiac rhythm disorder.

Symptom: Pain or pressure in the center of the chest or the arm or throat precipitated by exercise or following exercise (immediate or delayed).

Cause: Possible heart pain.

Remedy: Consult physician before resuming exercise program.

Symptom: Dizziness, lightheadedness, sudden uncoordination, confusion, cold sweat, glassy stare, pallor, blueness or fainting (immediate).

Cause: Insufficient blood to the brain.

Remedy: Do not try to cool down. Stop exercise and lie down with feet elevated, or put head down between legs until symptoms pass. Later consult physician before next exercise session.

Symptom: Persistent rapid heart action near the target level even five to ten minutes after the exercise was stopped (immediate).

Cause: Exercise is probably too vigorous.

Remedy: Keep heart rate at lower end of target zone or below. Increase the vigor of exercise more slowly. If these measures do not control the excessively high recovery heart rate, consult physician.

Symptom: Flare up of arthritic condition or gout which usually occurs in hips, knees, ankles, or big toe—the weight-bearing joints (immediate or delayed).

Cause: Trauma to joints which are particularly vulnerable.

Remedy: If you are familiar with how to quiet these flare-ups of your old joint condition, use your usual remedies. Rest up and do not resume your exercise program until the condition subsides. Then resume the exercise at a lower level with protective footwear or softer surfaces, or select other exercises which will put less strain on the imprired joints; e.g., swimming will be better for people with arthritis of the hips since it can be done mostly with the arms. If this is new arthritis, or if there is no response to usual remedies, see physician.

Symptom: Nausea or vomiting after exercise (immediate).
Cause: Not enough oxygen to the intestine. You are either exercising too vigorously or cooling down too quickly.
Remedy: Exercise less vigorously and be sure to take a more gradual and longer cooldown.

Symptom: Extreme breathlessness lasting more than ten minutes after stopping exercise (immediate).
Cause: Exercise is too taxing to your cardiovascular system or lungs.
Remedy: Stay at the lower end of your target range. If symptoms persist, do even less than target level. Be sure that while you are exercising you are not too breathless to talk to a companion.

Symptom: Prolonged fatigue even twenty-four hours later (delayed).
Cause: Exercise is too vigorous.
Remedy: Stay at lower end of target range or below. Increase level more gradually.

Symptom: Shinsplints—pain on the front or sides of lower leg) (delayed).
Cause: Inflammation of the fascia connecting the leg bones, or muscle tears where muscles of the lower leg connect to the bones.
Remedy: Use shoes with thicker soles. Work out in turf which is easier on your legs.

Symptom: Insomnia which was not present prior to the exercise program (delayed).
Cause: Exercise is too vigorous.
Remedy: Stay at lower end of target range or below. Increase intensity of exercise gradually.

Symptom: Pain in the calf muscles which occurs on heavy exercise but not at rest (immediate).

Cause: May be due to muscle cramps due to lack of use of these muscles, or exercising on hard surfaces. May also be due to poor circulation in the legs (called claudication).

Remedy: Use shoes with thicker soles, cooldown adequately. Muscle cramps should clear up after a few sessions. If "muscle cramps" do not subside, circulation is probably faulty. Try another type of exercise, e.g., bicycling instead of jogging in order to use different muscles.

Symptom: Side stitch—sticking under the ribs while exercising (immediate).

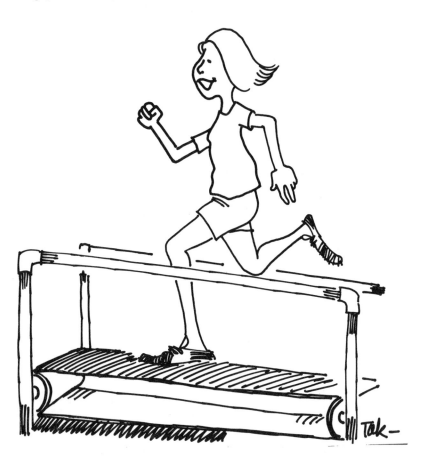

Cause: Diaphragm spasm. The diaphragm is the large muscle which separates the chest from the abdomen.

Remedy: Lean forward while sitting, attempting to push the abdominal organs up against the diaphragm.

Symptom: Charley horse or muscle-bound feeling (immediate or delayed).

Cause: Muscles are unconditioned and unaccustomed to exercise.

Remedy: Take hot bath and usual headache remedy. Next exercise should be less strenuous.

Source: *Beyond Diet: Exercise Your Way to Fitness and Heart Health* by Lenore R. Zohman, M.D., C.P.C. International, Englewood Cliffs, New Jersey. Single copies available gratis from: Mazola Oil Exercise Book, Department ZJH, Box 307, Coventry, Connecticut 06238.

BENEFITS OF TOTAL FITNESS
PHYSIOLOGICAL CHANGES

- aerobic exercise increases the total amount of blood in your system.
- the amount of oxygen—carrying hemoglobin in the blood is increased
- the working space and efficiency of the lungs increases
- heart and lung muscles become stronger, and with less effort work more efficiently
- ability to consume oxygen during strenuous exercise becomes far greater
- maximum working capacity and endurance dramatically increase
- resting heart rate is lower, less wear and tear on the heart
- muscle cells improve their ability to process oxygen and eliminate wastes more efficiently while requiring less blood blood
- skeletal muscles produce less lactic acid (by-product primarily responsible for feelings of fatigue)

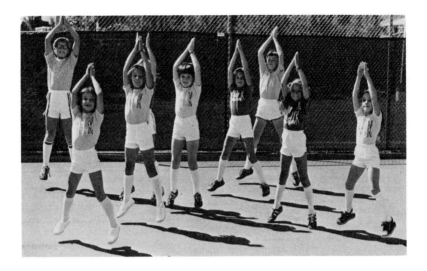

- blood vessels become more flexible, accumulating athero-sclerotic deposits much more slowly, yielding less work for the heart
- blood pressure, especially in hypertense individuals, is reduced
- the number of tiny blood vessels which form a network throughout the cells of the body are increased
- aerobic exercise tends to burn up the tensions of the day so that the body—chiefly the heart—can relax.
- after a cholesterol-rich meal, an aerobically trained person gets rid of the cholesterol more rapidly than the untrained
- aerobic exercise slightly lessens appetite
- aerobic exercise can and does result in substantial perma-nent weight loss
- muscles tone and firm through exercise
- weight loss lowers triglyceride levels
- weight reduction and exercise may lower uric acid levels
- exercise burns up both the fats in the blood and stored body fats
- blood chemistry is modified via raising the level of the small, protective, high-density lipoproteins (the "good guys" which carry cholesterol to the liver)
- blood chemistry is modified via lowering the number of dangerous low density lipoproteins (the "bad guys" that

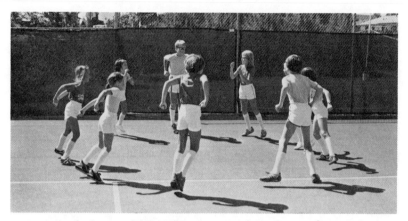

carry cholesterol into the tissues where it can form athero-sclerotic plaque which clogs up arteries and limits blood flow)

- aerobic exercise prevents or delays the onset of heart disease
- a fit body improves your chances of avoiding a heart attack
- having engaged in regular exercise will help you survive a heart attack if one does occur
- regular exercise helps to rehabilitate you following a heart attack

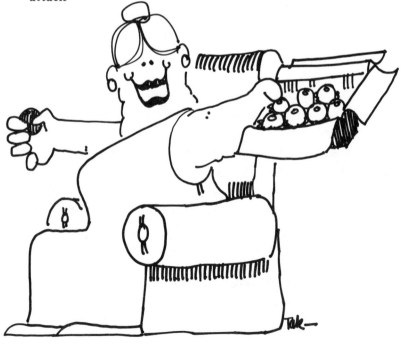

How to Calculate your Life Expectancy from How To by Peter Passell

No, we can't top Jeanne Dixon. But if you are between twenty and sixty-five and reasonably healthy, this test provides a life insurance company's eye-view of the future.

1. Start with seventy-two.

Gender

2. If you are male, subtract three. If you are female, add four. (That's right, there is a seven-year spread between the sexes).

Life Style

3. If you live in an urban area with a population over two million, subtract two. If you live in a town under ten thousand, or on a farm, add two. (City life means pollution, tension).

4. If you work behind a desk, subtract three. If your work requires regular, heavy physical labor, add three.

5. If you exercise strenuously (tennis, running, swimming, etc.) five times a week for at least one-half hour, add four. Two or three times a week, add two.

6. If you live with a spouse or friend, add five. If not, subtract one for every ten years alone since age twenty-five. (People together eat better, take care of each other, become less depressed).

Psyche

7. If you sleep more than ten hours each night, subtract four. (Excessive sleep is a sign of depression, circulatory diseases).

8. Are you intense, aggressive, easily angered? Subtract three. Are you easygoing, relaxed, a follower? Add three.

9. Are you happy? Add one. Unhappy? Subtract two.

10. Have you had a speeding ticket in the last year? Subtract one. (Accidents are the fourth largest cause of death; first, in young adults).

Success

11. Earn over $50,000 a year? Subtract two. (Wealth breeds high living, tension).

12. If you finished college, add one. If you have a graduate or professional degree, add two more. (Education seems to lead to moderation; at least that's the theory).

13. If you are sixty-five or over and still working, add three. (Retirement kills).

Heredity

14. If any grandparent lived to eighty-five, add two. If all four grandparents lived to eighty, add six.

15. If either parent died of a stroke or heart attack before the age of fifty, subtract four.

16. If any parent, brother, or sister under fifty has (or had) cancer or a heart condition, or has had diabetes since childhood, subtract three.

Health

17. Smoke more than two packs a day? Subtract eight. One to two packs? Subtract six. One-half to one? Subtract three.

18. Drink the equivalent of a quarter-bottle of liquor a day? Subtract one.

19. Overweight by fifty pounds or more? Subtract eight. Thirty to fifty pounds? Subtract four. Ten to thirty pounds? Subtract two.

20. Men over forty, if you have annual checkups, add two. Women, if you see a gynecologist once a year, add two.

Age Adjustment

21. Between thirty and forty? Add two. Between forty and fifty? Add three. Between fifty and seventy? Add four. Over seventy? Add five.

It's no fun playing the game unless you know how well you've done. The table below tells what percentage of the population you will outlive, providing you make it to the specified age.

Age	60	65	70	75	80	85	90	95	100
Men	26%	36%	48%	61%	75%	87%	96%	99%	99.6%
Women	15%	20%	30%	39%	53%	70%	88%	97%	99.6%

1.5 MILE RUN TEST
TIME (MINUTES)

Fitness Category

	Age (years) ►13-19		20-29	30-39
1. Very Poor	(men)	>15:31*	>16:01	>16:31
	(women)	>18:31	>19:01	>19:31
2. Poor	(men)	12:11-15:30	14:01-16:00	14:44-16:30
	(women)	18:30-16:55	19:00-18:31	19:30-19:01
3. Fair	(men)	10:49-12:10	12:01-14:00	12:31-14:45
	(women)	16:54-14:31	18:30-15:55	19:00-16:31
4. Good	(men)	9:41-10:48	10:46-12:00	11:01-12:30
	(women)	14:30-12:30	15:54-13:31	16:30-14:31
5. Excellent	(men)	8:37- 9:40	9:45-10:45	10:00-11:00
	(women)	12:29-11:50	13:30-12:30	14:30-13:00
6. Superior	(men)	< 8:37	< 9:45	< 10:00
	(women)	< 11:50	< 12:30	< 13:00

Fitness Category

	Age (years)► 40-49		50-59	60 +
1. Very Poor	(men)	>17:31	>19:01	>20:01
	(women)	>20:01	>20:31	>21:01
2. Poor	(men)	15:36-17:30	17:01-19:00	19:01-20:00
	(women)	20:00-19:31	20:30-20:01	21:00-21:31
3. Fair	(men)	13:01-15:35	14:31-17:00	16:16-19:00
	(women)	19:30-17:31	20:00-19:01	20:30-19:31
4. Good	(men)	11:31-13:00	12:31-14:30	14:00-16:15
	(women)	17:30-15:56	19:00-16:31	19:30-17:31
5. Excellent	(men)	10:30-11:30	11:00-12:30	11:15-13:59
	(women)	15:55-13:45	16:30-14:30	17:30-16:30
6. Superior	(men)	< 10:30	< 11:00	< 11:15
	(women)	< 13:45	< 14:30	< 16:30

* < Means "less than"; > Means "more than."

Six weeks of conditioning should precede this test. Take this test midway and at the end of the dance aerobics program. *Do not* take it until you are conditioned. Add thirty seconds for altitude of five to six thousand feet. Warm-up and cool down properly.

Source: From *The Aerobics Way* by Kenneth H. Cooper M.D., M.P.H. Copyright © 1977 by Kenneth H. Cooper. Reprinted by permission of the publisher, M. Evans and Company, New York, N.Y. 10017.

Bibliography

American College of Sports Medicine. *Guidelines for Graded Exercise Testing and Exercise Prescription.* Philadelphia: Lea & Febiger, 1975.

Anderson, Bobby. *Stretching.* Fullerton, California: By the Author, Box 2734, 1977.

Astrand, Per-orlof, and Rodahl, Kaare. *Textbook of Work Physiology.* New York: McGraw-Hill, 1977.

Bahr, Robert. "Can You Pass the Pinch Test?" *Runner's World,* January 1976, pp. 26-28.

Bird, Maureen, and Strobel, Joe. "How We Teach It." *Journal of Physical Education and Recreation,* June 1978, pp. 67-68.

Cendali, Richard. *Skip-It For Fun.* Boulder: Rocky Mountain Sports, 1977.

Clark, Matt, and Gosnell, Mariana. "How it Helps and Hurts." *Newsweek,* May 23, 1977, pp. 82-83.

Cooper, Kenneth, *Aerobics.* New York: Bantam Books, 1968.

Cooper, Kenneth. "How Aerobics Can Help Your Heart, and The Way You Feel." *Reader's Digest,* January 1978, pp. 117-121.

Cooper, Mildred, and Cooper, Kenneth. *Aerobics For Women.* New York: Bantam Books, 1973.

Cooper, Kenneth. *The Aerobics Way.* New York: M. Evans and Company, Inc., 1977.

Danford, Howard G.; Allen, Catherine L.; Dyer, Donald B.; Edgren, Harry D.; and Hjelte, George. *Goals for American Recreation.* Washington, D.C.: American Alliance for Health, Physical Education, Recreation, and Dance.

Edington, D.W., and Edgerton, V.R. *The Biology of Physical Activity.* Boston: Houghton-Mifflin Co., 1976.

Fales, E.D. "The Name of the Game is Health." *Parade,* September 15, 1974, p. 21.

Foster, Carl. "Physiological Requirements of Aerobic Dancing." *Research Quarterly* 46, March 1975, pp.120-122.

Friedman, Meyer, and Rosenman, Ray H. *Type A Behavior*

and Your Heart. Greenwich: Fawcett Publications, Inc., 1974.

Glass, David. "Stress, Competition, and Heart Attacks." *Psychology Today,* December 1976, pp. 54-57.

Glasser, William. *Positive Addiction.* New York: Harper & Row, 1976.

Gilmore, C.P. "Taking Exercise to Heart." *New York Times Magazine,* March 27, 1977, pp. 38-42.

Greenfield, Meg. "Two Cheers for the Unfit." *Newsweek,* January 2, 1978, p. 68.

Hanson, Kitty. *Disco Fever.* New York: New American Library, Inc., 1978.

H.E.W. "Fat People's Fight Against Job Bias: *U.S. News & World Report,* December 5, 1977, pp. 78-80.

Hursh, Lawrence. *Coronary Heart Disease: Risk Factors and the Diet Debate.* Chicago: National Dairy Council, 1975.

Johnson, Barry L., and Nelson, Jack K. *Practical Measurements for Evaluation in Physical Education.* Minneapolis: Burgess Publishing Company, 1974.

Kaplan, Janice. "The Aerobic Hustle." *Women's Sports,* December 1976.

Kreck, Carol. "Rhythm running—for the fun of it." *The Denver Post (Contemporary).* October 7, 1979, p. 8.

Lakat, Michael F. "In Pursuit of Hunger: Physiological Considerations." *Intellect,* February 1977, pp. 261-262.

Lang, John. "The Fitness Mania." *U.S. News & World Report,* February 27, 1978, pp. 37-40.

Meyer, H. *Old English Coffee Houses.* Emmaus, Pennsylvania: The Rodale Press, 1954.

Meyers, R.D. "Feeding Produced in the Satiated Rat." *Science,* June 9, 1972, pp. 1124-1125.

Polley, Maxine. "A Message From Dance Aerobics." *Journal of Physical Education and Recreation,* November-December 1978, p. 12.

Polley, Maxine. *Disco Basics.* Englewood Cliffs: Prentice-Hall, Inc., 1979.

Polley, Maxine. *Fitness: Dance Aerobics—Secondary Routines.* Fort Collins: Robinson Press, 1978. (out of print).

Rosenfield, Paul. "Cooper's Cohorts Run Down Heart Disease." *Saturday Evening Post,* September 1977, pp. 18-20.

Schuster, Karolyn. "Aerobic Dance: A Step to Fitness." *The Physician & Sportsmedicine,* August, 1979, pp. 98-103.

Sorensen, Neil. Personal letter of September 28, 1979.

Strecker, E.A. and Chambers, F.T. *Alcohol: One Man's Meat.* New York: The Macmillan Co., 1978, p. 38.

Time. "Perrier Survey of Fitness in America," February 5, 1979, p. 140.

Time. "Ready, Set, Sweat," June 6, 1977, pp. 82-83.

Ukers, W.H. *All About Coffee.* New York: The Tea & Coffee Trade Journal Co., 1935, p. 314.

Van Doorn, John. "An Intimidating New Class: The Physical Elite." *New York,* May 29, 1978.

Vannier, Maryhelen. *Recreation Leadership.* Philadelphia: Lea & Febiger, 1977.

Waters, Harry; Whitman, Lisa; Martin, Ann; and Gram, Dewey. "Keeping Fit: America Tries to Shape Up." *Newsweek,* May 23, 1977, pp. 78-83.

Weiner, Bob. "Disco Sally Struts Her Stuff." *New York.* May 29, 1978, pp. 56-57.

Zinman, David. "Competition Among The Kids." *Runner's World,* January 1977, pp. 24-25.

Zohman, Lenore. *Exercise Your Way to Fitness and Heart Health.* Englewood Cliffs: C.P.C. International, Inc., 1974.

Zohman, Lenore R.; Kattus, Albert A.; and Softness, Donald G. *The Cardiologists' Guide to Fitness and Health Through Exercise.* New York: Simon and Schuster, 1979.

About the Author

Maxine Polley is an author, the dance aerobics instructor at Colorado State University (DCE), and a Clinician on the Colorado Governor's Council for Health Promotion and Physical Fitness.

She attributes her early cardiovascular fitness to acrobatic and rhythms training begun at age five, six years at Dotty Stuart McGill's School of Dance, marching five years with the National Champion Plaidettes Drill Team, and touring United States and Canada with the Lucky Girls Acrobatic Team.

Valedictorian of her high school, cum laude graduate of Slippery Rock State College, Maxine received her Masters in Physical Education and has completed the doctoral coursework at the University of Northern Colorado, Greeley.

She is most proud of her children—Rex (12), Dee (10), Dana (9), and neighborhood youngsters who perform as the Aerobic Angels. Maxine and her husband, Dr. Dale Polley, Director of Special Education Services of Poudre R-1 Schools, reside with their children in Fort Collins, Colorado.

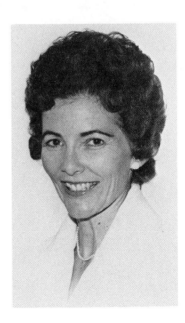

About the Illustrator

Sharon Waag received her B.A. and M.A. in Fine Arts and Elementary Education from the University of Northern Colorado. She taught first grade at Bedford, Iowa, and art education in Windsor and LaPorte, Colorado, at the elementary level.

A true homemaker, she discontinued teaching professionally when her first child was born. While illustrating books as a hobby, her two youngsters, Lynette (17), and Steven (15), kept her constantly challenged and happy.

Now Sharon is employed along with her husband, Harold, at the Woodward Governor Company in Fort Collins. The family resides in Timnath, Colorado.

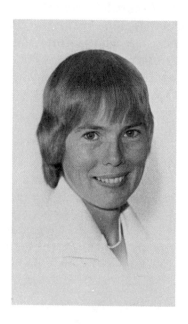